Dr. AI - The Future Of Medicine?

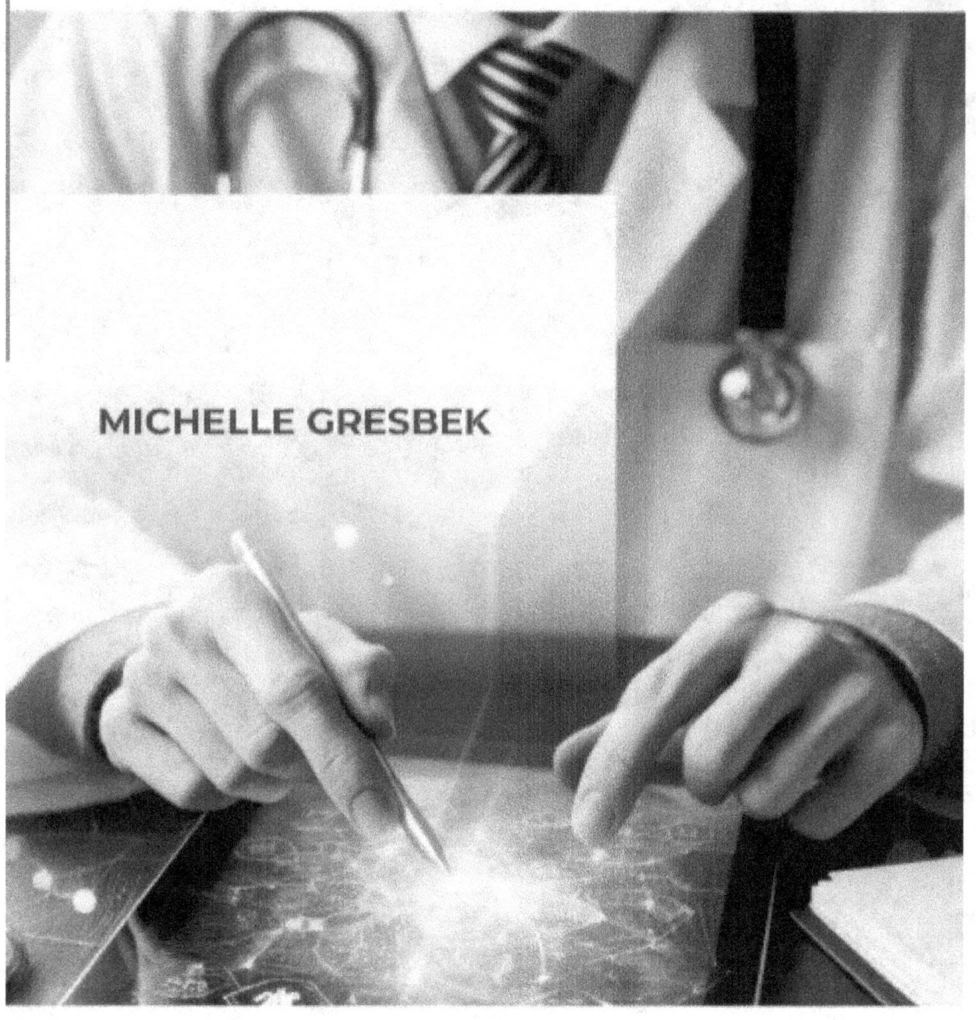

MICHELLE GRESBEK

© 2024

Preface

In her captivating new book "Dr. AI - The Future Of Medicine?" Michelle Gresbek takes us on a journey through the exciting world of Artificial Intelligence (AI) and its groundbreaking influence on medicine. The book provides a deep insight into the fundamentals, challenges, and potentials that the integration of AI applica-

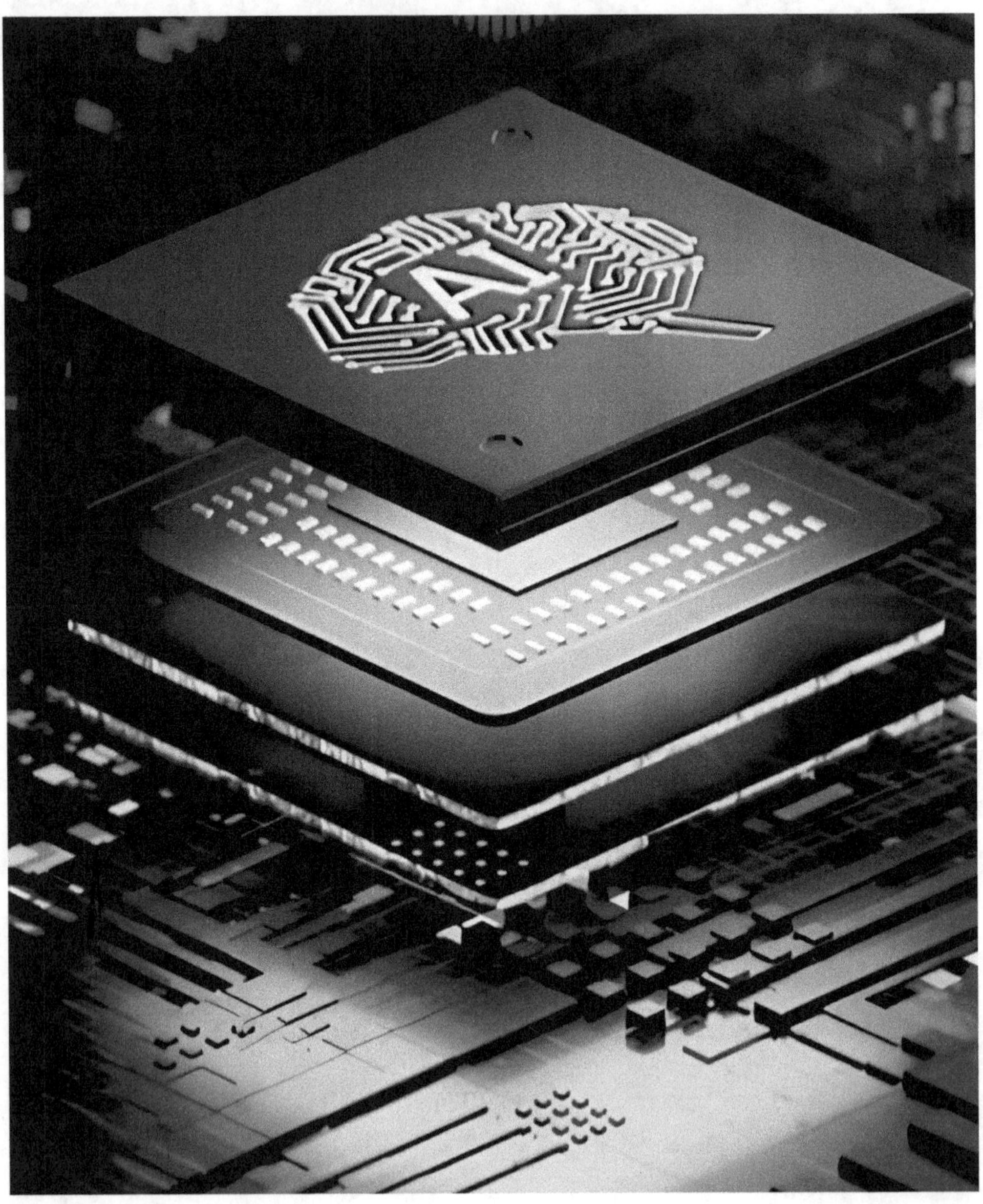

tions brings to the healthcare sector. In a time where technological progress and ethical questions intersect, Michelle Gresbek navigates through this complex terrain, delivering a comprehensive overview of the historical development, economic significance, and strategic relevance of Artificial Intelligence.

The author not only illuminates the technical prerequisites and ethical principles but also discusses the legal framework crucial for the successful implementation of AI in healthcare. She emphasizes the importance of digital competence, professional qualifications, and transparency as key aspects to promote the integration of AI in healthcare.

Throughout the book, concrete examples of AI applications in healthcare are presented. From medical chatbots to early diagnostics and the detection and management of pandemics, Michelle Gresbek provides a clear insight into the enormous potential that AI holds for the future of medicine. The book critically analyzes not only the opportunities but also the risks of this technology, especially concerning the potential misuse of health data, misinterpretations, and the limitation of interaction between doctors and patients.

"Dr. AI - The Future Of Medicine?" is an essential work that introduces not only healthcare professionals but also readers without a medical background to the fascinating world of Artificial Intelligence. It offers a holistic view of the transformation of medicine through innovative technologies and encourages a thoughtful engagement with the challenges and opportunities involved.

Content

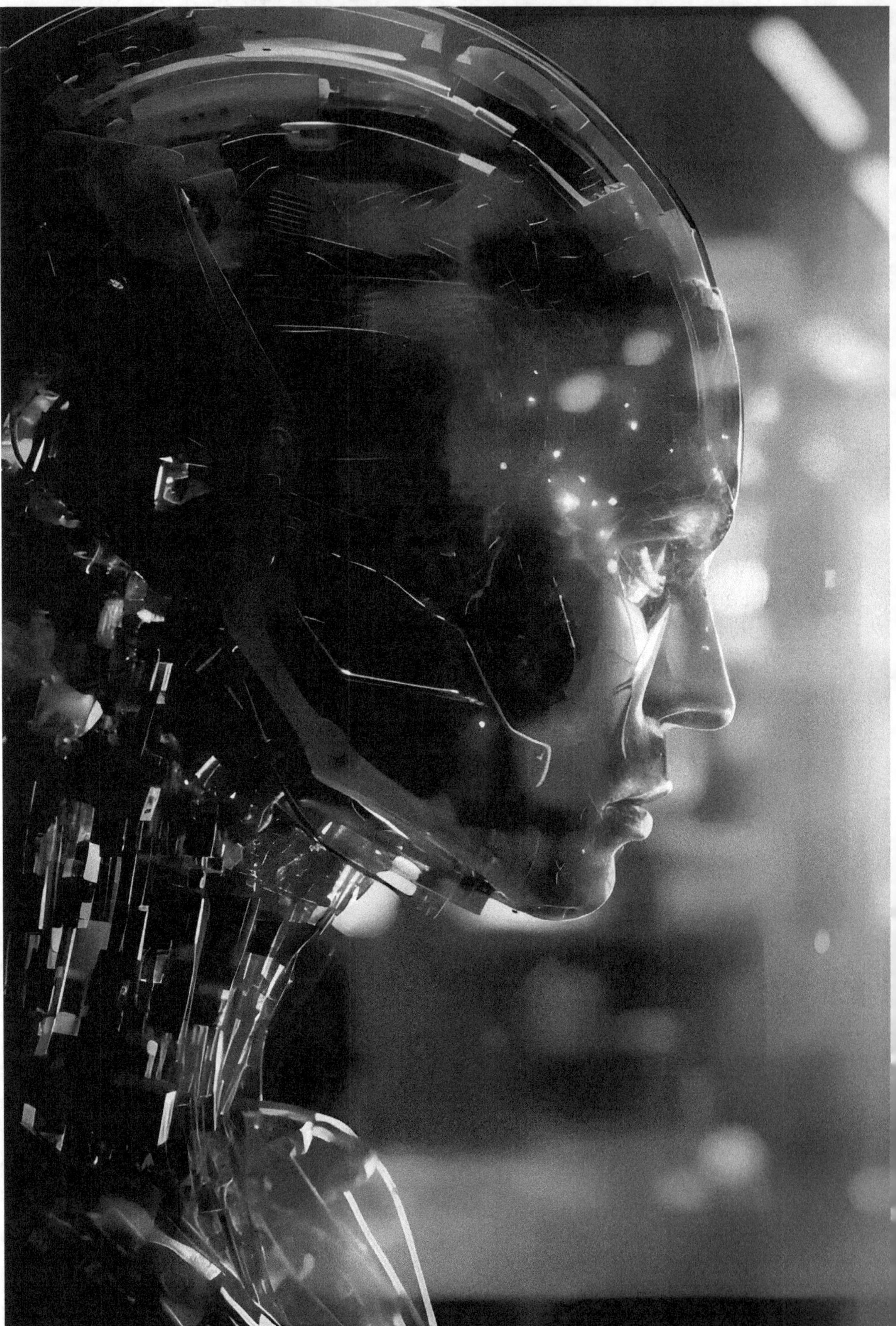

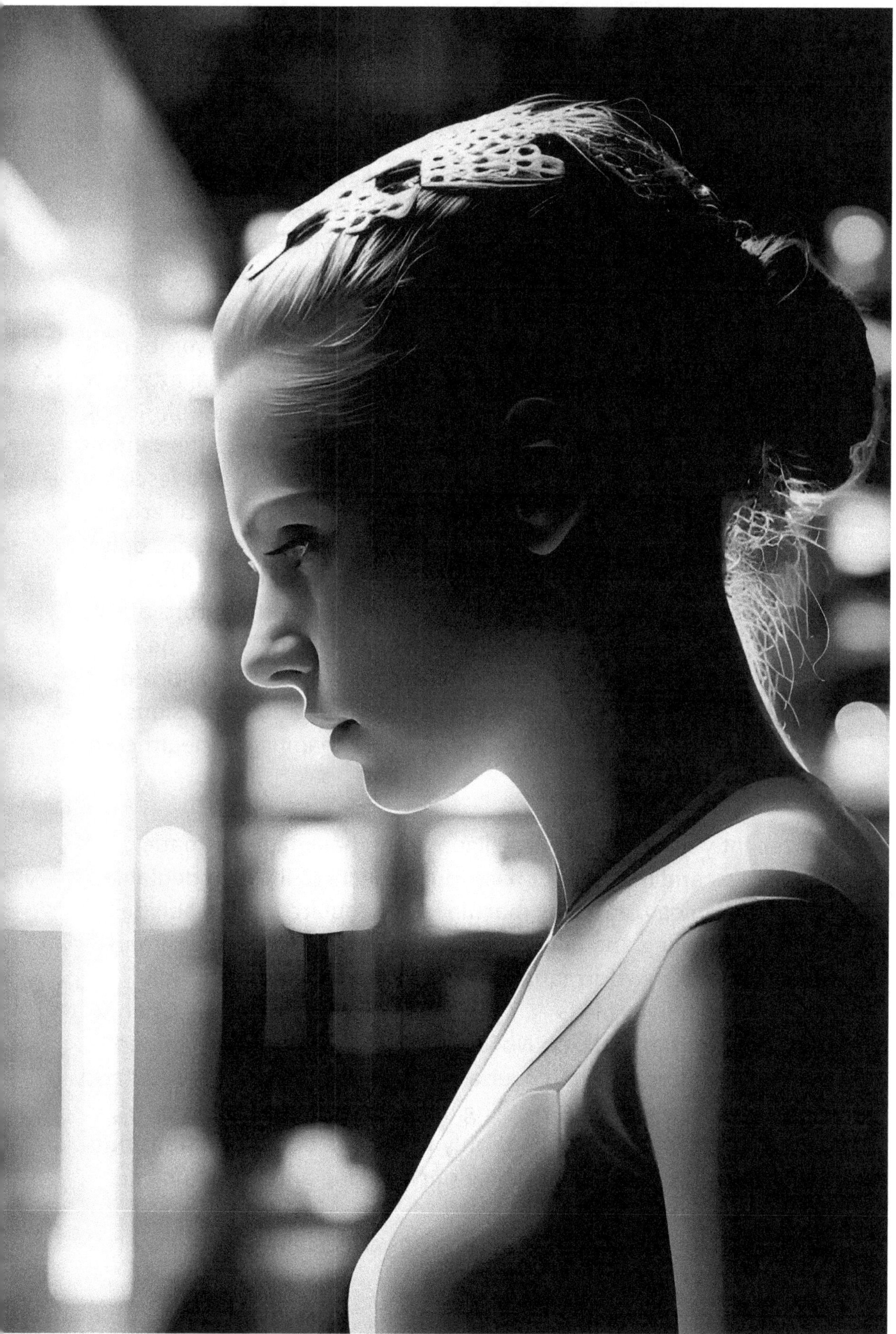

1 Introduction

The rapid development of Artificial Intelligence (AI) in recent years has initiated a remarkable transformation in various aspects of life. This technology enables machines to simulate human abilities such as learning and understanding. A standout example of this development is "ChatGPT," a novel and publicly accessible tool from the technology company OpenAI, released on November 30, 2022. Within just five days of its release, it gained global attention and already had over a million users. The increasing popularity of AI technologies illustrates their enormous potential to fundamentally change our thinking and behavior. This book takes a fascinating look into the world of Artificial Intelligence, particularly in the context of its application in the healthcare sector. It not only highlights the opportunities but also explores potential risks and challenges to provide a balanced perspective on the future of this revolutionary technology. In a time where at least 5% of the total expenditures in the medical sector are expected to be allocated to Artificial Intelligence, it becomes evident that the decisions we make today will lay the foundation for shaping the healthcare landscape of tomorrow.

In recent years, Artificial Intelligence (AI) has made dramatic advances, and its impact on various aspects of life is undeniable. This technology, enabling machines to simulate human abilities such as learning and understanding, is at the center of a remarkable societal transformation. An outstanding example of AI's influence on daily life is "ChatGPT," an innovative tool by OpenAI released to the public on November 30, 2022. It quickly gained global attention and had over a million users. The rising popularity of ChatGPT reflects the growing importance of AI technologies, which have the potential not only to change our interactions but also to fundamentally influence our thinking and behavior.

However, this development also raises critical questions, especially regarding the potential impact of AI on various aspects of life. The focus is not only on the opportunities but also on the challenges and potential risks. This book emphasizes the application of AI in the healthcare sector, a field that is particularly scrutinized due to its high individual and societal significance. Since its initial steps in the 1990s, the significance of AI applications in healthcare has significantly increased. Predictions suggest that in the near future, at least 5% of the total expenditures in the medical sector could be allocated to Artificial Intelligence. In this dynamic interplay between opportunities and risks, it is crucial to find a balanced path and shape the developments in AI responsibly.

Neural networks like ChatGPT are based on supervised learning and reinforcement learning, allowing them to respond to a wide range of topics with sufficient accuracy. Studies have shown that ChatGPT, although not specialized in medicine, is capable of providing diagnoses in the emergency room at least as accurately as doctors. In some cases, the "Chatbot" even outperformed the doctors, but it was noted that it is also prone to errors. In another study, Artificial Intelligence competed against 118 pulmonologists evaluating a lung function test. The algorithm accurately assessed 82% of all cases within a short time, while the pulmonologists had correctly evaluated only about 45%

These studies demonstrate that Artificial Intelligence is capable of, among other things, detecting diseases early, supporting diagnoses, personalizing therapies, assisting in surgeries, accelerating research, and analyzing health data. On the other hand, risks associated with Artificial Intelligence must not be overlooked. It is crucial to analyze and communicate both the potentials and risks of AI to ensure responsible utilization.

This book provides a comprehensive insight into this topic, discussing how the decisions made today will significantly influence the healthcare landscape of tomorrow.

2. Fundamentals

The current era, characterized by rapid technological advancements and societal transformations, may be on the verge of another epochal moment that will fundamentally reshape civilization. A retrospective look into recent history reveals that the introduction of machines and the utilization of steam and later electricity not only revolutionized production methods but also led to profound societal changes. Another milestone in human history is the rapid development of computer technology and the establishment of the internet in the 20th century.

These technologies have revolutionized the way we communicate, share information, and work. The interconnection of computers and the creation of a global information network have ushered the world into an era of digitization that influences nearly every aspect of our daily lives. Simultaneously, a global pandemic, dynamic changes in supply chains, and unexpected geopolitical conflicts have created new challenges. Amidst these new demands, Artificial Intelligence plays a central role. The utilization of AI is made possible by advanced data infrastructure and computing power, and the focus has shifted from simple AI implementation to realizing values and fully harnessing its potential.

Similar to the groundbreaking changes in agriculture and electricity, we are now experiencing a new phase of transformation driven by Artificial Intelligence. In 2023, a groundbreaking innovation was presented to the public – an autonomously learning application capable of communicating on par with humans. This advanced chatbot marks another step in the dynamic evolution of technologies and underscores the ongoing revolution propelled by Artificial Intelligence.

Sundar Pichai, CEO of Google, emphasizes that Artificial Intelligence will be as powerful or dangerous as human nature allows, and that the upcoming revolution will be faster and more extensive than many people can imagine. This moment of upheaval challenges humanity to explore the impacts and potentials of AI comprehensively and critically, ensuring an informed and responsible use of this technology.

2.1 Definitions and Historical Development:

The term "Artificial Intelligence" (AI) first emerged in the 1950s when John McCarthy, a U.S. computer scientist, used it in a project proposal to the Rockefeller Foundation. AI refers to technologies that aim to perform tasks that typically require human intelligence. Defining AI proves challenging as terms like "intelligence" and "intelligent human behavior" themselves are not fully defined. Nevertheless, the functioning of AI technology is modeled on processes resembling the human brain. AI enables systems to learn from experiences and data to improve their performance and capabilities over time. Unlike traditional computer programs, AI applications learn without explicit programming for a task.

Kaplan and Haenlein (2019) define AI as the ability of a system to interpret external data, learn from it, and adapt insights flexibly to achieve specific goals and tasks. AI is an interdisciplinary concept that seeks to mimic human intelligence by having algorithms comprehend complex ideas and solve problems. Within AI, there are subfields such as Machine Learning (ML), where Neural Networks (NN) and Deep Learning (DL) represent specific methods.

Machine Learning is a subfield of AI that develops systems capable of learning from data, recognizing patterns, and making predictions. Neural networks, inspired by the structure of the human brain, are computer models within the field of machine learning. Deep Learning is a specific manifestation of machine learning based on multi-layered artificial neural networks. The challenge lies in the fact that the performance of Deep Learning heavily depends on the availability of large amounts of training data. The terms AI, Machine Learning, and Deep Learning should not be used synonymously; AI is the overarching term, while ML represents a specific technique, and DL is a particular method within ML.

In the discussion of Artificial Intelligence, a distinction is made between weak AI and strong AI. Strong AI aims to replicate human functions, while weak AI is capable of fulfilling well-defined tasks but is limited to a single task. The introduction of "Large Language Models (LLMs)" has brought AI into the public consciousness. These powerful models can process natural language and generate complex texts. The development of these chatbots began in 2018 with GPT-1, followed by GPT-2 and the groundbreaking GPT-3 and GPT-3.5. Currently, GPT-4 and ChatGPT Plus are relevant, with GPT-4V (GPT-4 Vision) representing a significant advancement as a large multimodal model capable of understanding not only text but also images and videos.

2.1.1 How does ChatGPT work?

The core of ChatGPT is a Large Language Model ("LLM"), or a large language model. The current LLM for ChatGPT is GPT-3.5 or GPT-4. A large language model is a neural network-based model trained on massive amounts of text data to understand and generate human language. The model uses training data to learn the statistical patterns and relationships between words in the language, then utilizes this knowledge to predict the subsequent words, one word at a time. An LLM is often characterized by its size and the number of parameters it contains. The largest model of GPT-3.5 has 175 billion parameters distributed across 96 layers in the neural network, making it one of the largest deep learning models ever created. The model's input and output are organized into tokens. Tokens are numerical representations of words or, more precisely, parts of words. Numbers are used for tokens instead of words because they can be processed more efficiently. GPT-3.5 was trained on a large dataset of internet data, with the source dataset containing 500 billion tokens. In other words, the model was trained on hundreds of billions of words. The model was trained to predict the next token in a sequence of input tokens. It can generate text structured in a way that is grammatically correct and semantically similar to the internet data on which it was trained.

However, without proper guidance, the model can also generate outputs that are incorrect, toxic, or reflect harmful sentiments. Despite this significant drawback, the model can be "trained" to perform natural language tasks using carefully constructed text prompts. This is where the new field of "Prompt Engineering" comes into play.

To make the model safer, it is further fine-tuned through a process called Reinforcement Learning from Human Feedback (RLHF).

In March 2023, OpenAI released its GPT-4 model for paying subscribers of ChatGPT Plus. This innovation marks a significant advancement in ChatGPT's capabilities, especially in handling complex tasks. At the same time, it reflects OpenAI's efforts to reduce undesired or harmful responses.

The most significant change from GPT-3.5 to GPT-4 lies in the context window, which expanded from about 3,000 words at the release of ChatGPT to approximately 25,000 for GPT-4. Additionally, the model now produces more accurate information, exhibits fewer hallucinations, and responds less frequently to sensitive requests or generates unauthorized content.

Another notable improvement is GPT-4's ability to accept image inputs, although it can only generate text responses. However, the next product from OpenAI takes multimodality to a new level.

Released in July 2023, the Code Interpreter is OpenAI's latest AI system as of August 2023. It is based on the GPT-4 model but brings significant enhancements.

Most notably, its ability to understand inputs and generate outputs in multiple formats (text, image, video, audio, code) exponentially increases its capability to comprehend information and produce desired results.

ChatGPT became a global cultural phenomenon almost overnight, achieving unprecedented mainstream popularity. OpenAI leveraged this momentum to release fine-tuned versions of ChatGPT and new models more rapidly.

The GPT technology has now reached its peak—not in terms of its capabilities (the limitations are numerous) but in terms of people's expectations.

In a conversation with the MIT Technology Review, the OpenAI team revealed how they are working to improve ChatGPT.

A significant issue is Jailbreaking, which involves tricking ChatGPT to provide restricted information. The OpenAI team is attempting to teach the AI system to ignore such requests through adversarial training. This involves pitting two chatbots against each other, with one trying to get the other to bypass its limitations. The resulting outputs serve as training data for ChatGPT.

Another major issue with GPT models is factual accuracy. Every AI tool is only as good as the data it was trained on. The selection of training data is a delicate matter and a crucial factor in the model's performance. Factual accuracy is likely to remain an issue, and anyone using ChatGPT and similar technologies should be aware of this.

Although GPT-4 emerged shortly after the launch of ChatGPT, there are already rumors about GPT-5. OpenAI even filed a trademark application for GPT-5 in July 2023—currently under review by the United States Patent and Trademark Office (USPTO). However, OpenAI CEO Sam Altman stated that the company is not currently working on the next model and has no timeline for its release. He emphasized the need to address security issues beforehand.

ChatGPT has forever changed the AI landscape. It sparked increased interest in natural language processing, leading to a wave of research and accelerated technological development. The market is flooded with AI solutions, and many companies have integrated ChatGPT into their workflows.

2.1.2 The Most Important "Generative AI Companies" and Their Focus Areas

The world of Generative Artificial Intelligence is significantly shaped by a few leading companies focusing on different areas. These companies set groundbreaking standards and crucially influence the development and application of Generative AI. In this overview, we take a brief look at the most significant "Generative AI Companies" and their respective focus areas, shaping the future of this innovative technology.

OpenAI: Best Overall Performance

OpenAI is considered the most successful Generative AI company with an estimated valuation of around 29 billion US dollars. It offers products like GPT-3, GPT-4, ChatGPT Plus, DALL-E, and Whisper. Despite its financial strength, OpenAI is occasionally criticized for generating inaccurate or even offensive content.

Hugging Face: Focus on Community-Driven AI Development

Hugging Face stands out as a platform for community-driven AI development, enabling developers to create and optimize their own Generative AI solutions. Partnerships with AWS and the integration of Hugging Face products into the cloud sector strengthen its position.

Alphabet (Google): Focus on Scalability

Google, a subsidiary of Alphabet, leads in AI scalability. With a focus on cloud ecosystems, Google integrates Generative AI support into various applications. Comprehensive AI ethics principles and a relatively transparent approach aim to further solidify its market position.

Microsoft: Focus on Business Operations and Productivity

Microsoft, with a market valuation of 2.25 trillion US dollars, is a dynamic player in the field of Generative AI. By developing its own tools and supporting OpenAI innovations, such as Copilot, Microsoft provides solutions for business operations and productivity.

Cohere: Focus on Natural Language Processing (NLP)

Cohere stands out with its advanced NLP tools enabling text search, classification, and generation. With products like Neural Search, Summarize, and Generate, Cohere facilitates the customization of AI models to specific business requirements.

Anthropic: Focus on Customizable Content

Anthropic focuses on high-quality and secure content development through products like Claude. It is highly customizable and finds applications in customer service, legal matters, office administration, and sales.

Jasper: Focus on Marketers

Jasper offers generative AI solutions for marketers, with features supporting blog and email writing, SEO optimization, and image generation. Its brand alignment and user-friendly interface strengthen its position in the market.

Glean: Focus on Employee User Experience

Glean provides generative AI-supported internal search for workplace apps and ecosystems. Companies can use Glean to facilitate the search for corporate knowledge and tailor information to employees' specific roles.

Synthesis AI: Focus on a Variety of Generative AI Use Cases

Synthesis AI distinguishes itself with a wide range of products for synthetic data, image, and video generation. Applications range from identity verification to 3D human modeling, strengthened by a commitment to AI ethics and diversity.

Stability AI: Focus on Foundation for Other Generative AI Solutions

Stability AI focuses on providing a foundation for other Generative AI solutions. With an emphasis on stability and security, the company offers technologies that can serve as a basis for the development of more advanced Generative AI solutions.

These companies profoundly influence the world of Generative Artificial Intelligence by setting standards and crucially shaping the development and application of this innovative technology. Each company has its unique focus areas, contributing to shaping the future of Generative AI.

Stability AI provides the foundation for many innovative Generative AI solutions. With the Stable Diffusion 2.0 model and an extensive API library, it offers an open platform for developers, although it faces profitability issues and controversies.

Lightricks: Focus on Personal and Creative Use

Lightricks, renowned for its photo editing apps, has successfully ventured into generative AI with text-to-image functionality. While less relevant for business applications, it provides user-friendly tools for creative use.

Inflection AI: Focus on Visionary Outlook

Inflection AI looks somewhat different from the other top Generative AI companies on this list as it has not yet released any products.

2.2 Economic and Strategic Significance of Artificial Intelligence

Artificial Intelligence is poised to become a significant economic factor. According to projections from the McKinsey Global Institute (MGI), an average increase of 1.2 percentage points in Gross Domestic Product (GDP) per year is expected through AI by 2030. This surpasses the economic impact of historical innovations such as the steam engine, industrial robots, and information and communication technologies by a considerable margin.

The steam engine contributed to a 0.3 percentage point increase in GDP, industrial robots added 0.4 percentage points, and information and communication technologies saw a rise of 0.6 percentage points.

2.2.1 Importance for the Gross National Product of Leading Nations

Before the COVID-19 crisis, it was estimated that the global AI market would reach a value of around $90 billion by 2025. Of this, the United States was expected to account for $43 billion, Europe for an additional $20 billion, and China anticipated a revenue of $52 billion by 2025. PricewaterhouseCoopers (PwC) predicts that Germany's Gross Domestic Product could increase by 9.9% by 2030 thanks to AI.

AI offers opportunities ranging from creating new jobs to optimizing processes and developing entirely new business models. Companies strategically leveraging AI have the chance to strengthen their competitiveness and explore new markets.

This technology plays a crucial role in shaping the future global economy.

2.2.2 AI's Strategic Influence and Economic Contributions to Healthcare

Global superpowers have developed comprehensive strategies to promote Artificial Intelligence. China aims to be a global leader in AI by 2030. Europe has an EU AI strategy, and in 2021, the EU Commission proposed the world's first legal framework for AI. AI already plays a significant role in the European healthcare sector.
McKinsey studies indicate that around 56% of healthcare professionals have experience with AI. The implementation of AI is expected to replace a substantial share of working hours by 2030. In the healthcare sector, AI will contribute to making existing healthcare professionals more efficient by deploying human empathy where it is most crucial, while AI-assisted systems take on tasks related to data analysis and management.

2.3 Overview of Artificial Intelligence in Healthcare

The use of Artificial Intelligence is gaining increasing importance in the field of medicine, finding application in various areas, including research, education, early detection, diagnosis, therapy, and care.

The medical field has seen the highest growth in scientific publications on the use of AI. According to the PubMed database, the number of scientific articles on AI in medicine has increased from about 2,000 in 2018 to over 12,000 in 2021.

The predicted increase in scientific publications underscores the expectation of significant research breakthroughs attributed to the use of AI in science. The delivery of high-quality healthcare in the future is expected to depend significantly on AI-based applications, as modern medicine becomes increasingly complex.

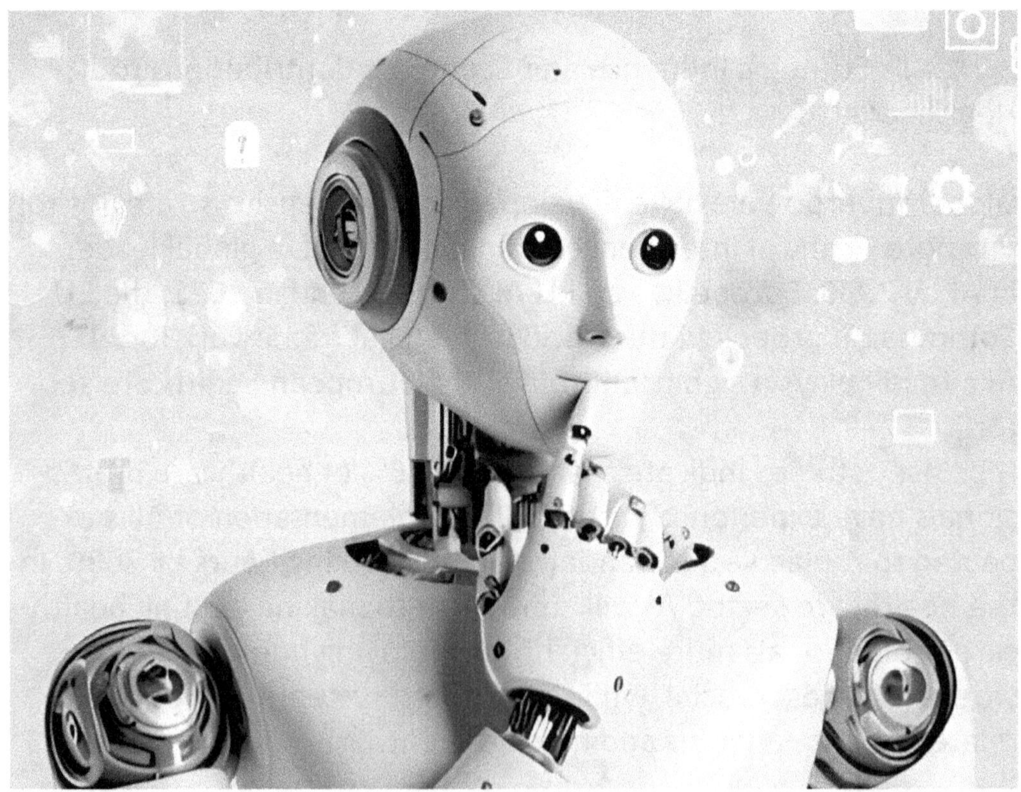

Within the healthcare domain, the deployment of Artificial Intelligence (AI) transcends traditional boundaries, encompassing a spectrum of applications that range from the development of digital companions and early warning systems to the creation of sophisticated diagnostic tools, personalized therapy options, and innovative care robots.

AI's intrinsic ability to process and analyze various types of data opens up a plethora of diverse application areas, contributing significantly to the enhancement of healthcare services. This extensive scope includes delivering personalized health information tailored to individual needs, facilitating early detection of diseases, employing advanced diagnostic algorithms for medical images, and providing insightful interpretations of clinical findings. The multifaceted applications of AI in healthcare not only streamline processes but also pave the way for groundbreaking advancements in personalized medicine, patient care, and overall healthcare management.

AI can create and monitor personalized therapy plans, support the management and monitoring of patients in healthcare, automate rehabilitation after injuries or surgeries, and simplify administrative tasks such as appointment scheduling and billing. Furthermore, AI plays a role in the education and training of healthcare personnel, accelerates medical research through the analysis of large datasets, and contributes to improving public health.

This includes better monitoring of epidemics or pandemics and supporting healthcare prevention. In detail, chatbots can capture symptoms and provide treatment recommendations, AI-assisted image recognition can identify malignant tumor cells, voice recordings can be examined for early signs of dementia, and AI can support healing processes as well as the planning of rehabilitation measures. Robotics is also gaining importance and is increasingly being used in nursing, logistics, and the operating room.

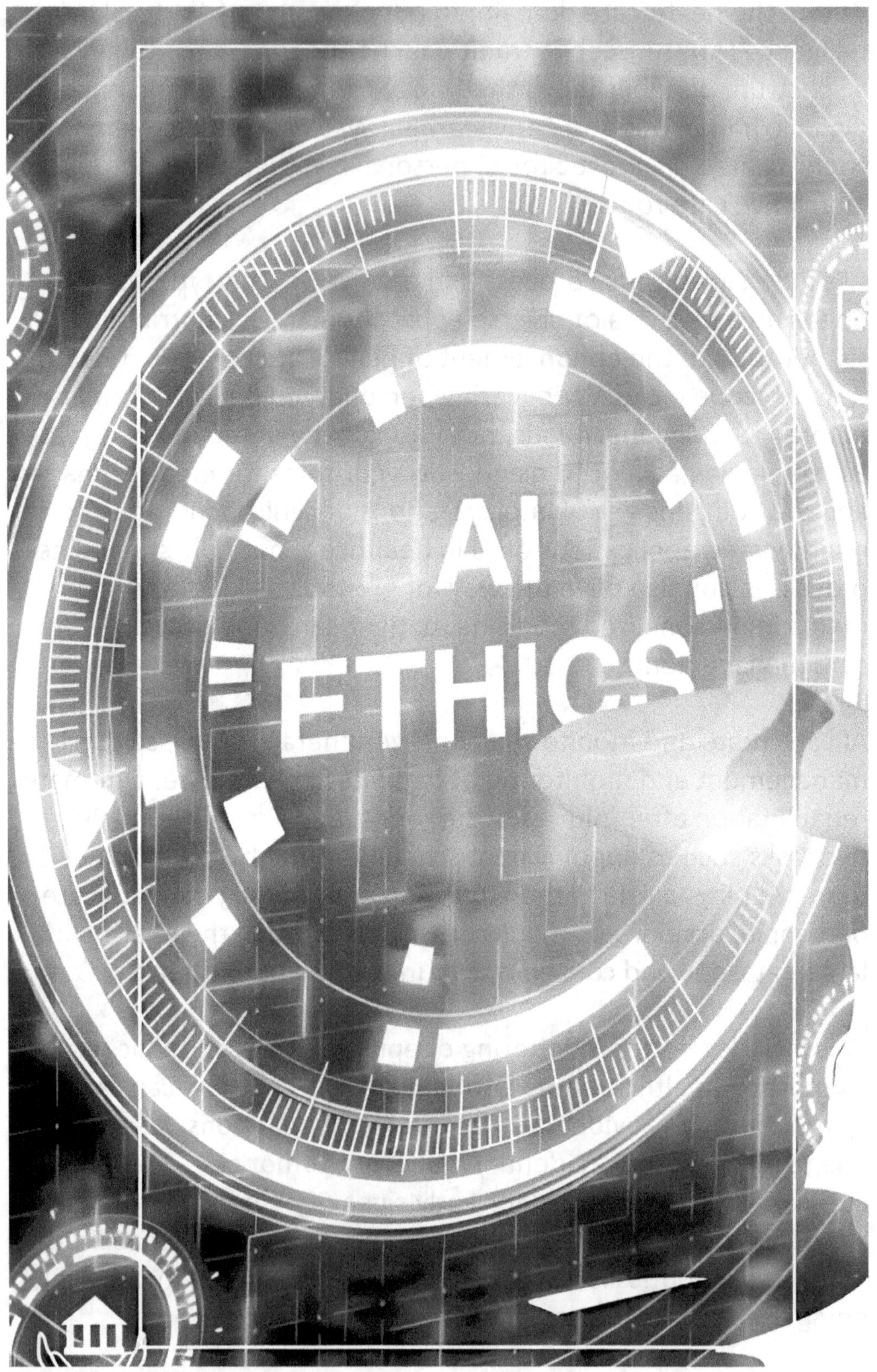

AI
ETHICS

3. Conditions and Requirements for AI Implementation

With the rapid progress of Artificial Intelligence (AI), it is becoming increasingly crucial to establish not only technical but also ethical and legal frameworks to ensure the safe and responsible use of this technology. These measures are essential to foster societal trust in AI applications, especially in the healthcare sector.

3.1 Technical Prerequisites

The technical conditions for the implementation of Artificial Intelligence have undergone significant developments in recent decades. While the theoretical foundations of intelligent systems existed, the available computing power of computers was insufficient for demanding tasks for a long time. Advances in storage capacities and computing power, especially through graphic processors, have overcome these hurdles. However, the limited availability of high-quality datasets, particularly in Germany, remains a central challenge and a potential impediment to innovation.

3.2 Clarification of Ethical Principles

Important steps towards a common good-oriented regulation of Artificial Intelligence (AI) have already been taken. Nevertheless, there is substantial need for action to address the challenges in the field of AI in line with ethical principles and human rights.

Questions that need to be addressed include:

- Transparency and Explainability: How can AI systems be designed to be transparent, and how can decisions made by AI systems be made understandable for humans?

- Non-discrimination: How can it be ensured that AI systems do not promote discrimination based on gender, race, religion, or other characteristics?

- Privacy and Data Protection: What measures can be taken to protect the privacy of users and ensure that personal data is handled appropriately?

- Security and Robustness: How can the security of AI systems be ensured, and how can they be protected against unwanted influences or attacks?

- Accountability: Who is responsible for the decisions and actions of AI systems, and how can liability be regulated in case of malfunctions?

- Participation and Inclusion: How can various interest groups be involved in the development process of AI to ensure that different perspectives are considered?

- Long-term Impacts: What potential long-term impacts can be attributed to the widespread application of AI technologies on society, employment, and the economy?

- Cultural Diversity: How can AI systems respect cultural diversity and appropriately consider different social and cultural contexts?

- Education and Access: How can it be ensured that the benefits of AI technologies are distributed fairly, and that education and access to these technologies are accessible to all?

- Ethical Research: What ethical principles should be considered in AI research to ensure that it respects and promotes societal values?

These questions represent only a fraction of the complex ethical considerations arising in connection with the development and application of AI.

With the rapid progress of Artificial Intelligence, it is becoming increasingly crucial to establish not only technical but also ethical and legal frameworks to ensure a safe and responsible use of this technology. These measures are essential to foster societal trust in AI applications, especially in the healthcare sector.

A milestone in this context is the "Recommendation on the Ethics of Artificial Intelligence," adopted by the 193 UNESCO member states in November 2021. This groundbreaking recommendation establishes clear guidelines for the ethical development and use of AI, covering eleven policy areas.

The recommendation provides an essential framework for the responsible development and utilization of AI technologies. It reflects the aspiration to place ethical principles and human rights at the forefront of AI unfolding. The eleven policy areas covered by the recommendation include various aspects such as education, culture, communication, labor, and health. This broad coverage illustrates that the ethical development and use of AI have far-reaching impacts on different aspects of life and must be considered comprehensively.

The "Recommendation on the Ethics of Artificial Intelligence" not only sets clear standards for the industry but also creates an international framework aiming to positively shape the societal impacts of AI. It not only calls for compliance with ethical principles but also establishes clear mandates for the governments of UNESCO member states. This is intended to ensure that AI technologies are regulated worldwide in a manner consistent with human rights and the common good.
Overall, the "Recommendation on the Ethics of Artificial Intelligence" marks a significant step toward global governance of AI.

It emphasizes the urgency of placing ethical principles and human rights at the center of AI development and provides a framework for coordinated international efforts to collectively shape the given challenges and opportunities.

3.3 Establishment of Legal Frameworks

The challenge for national governments is to find balanced regulations for Artificial Intelligence (AI) that do not hinder innovation. A balanced approach is required to ensure the acceptance of new technologies while establishing clear frameworks for businesses and protective mechanisms for consumers. National interests, particularly efforts for economic dominance and protection in global competition, complicate the search for a global consensus.

In the United States, there was initially no federal AI legislation. However, with an Executive Order from President Joe Biden, a framework was created to protect national security and citizens' rights. Rules for the development and marketing of AI tools are introduced, security test results must be shared, and standards for the safety of AI solutions are developed. The Executive Order emphasizes the protection of citizens' rights and the prevention of societal conflicts caused by AI models.

China's regulatory approach to Artificial Intelligence is characterized by two main aspects. On the one hand, it is strongly innovation-oriented, with initiatives to promote specific developments being driven at various levels of government and industry. On the other hand, the approach is socially oriented, with "social stability" taking precedence over an individual's rights, according to the understanding of the central government. It is emphasized that despite promoting innovation, social harmony and stability are considered overarching goals. However, the current draft law in China also indicates that certain regulations propose stricter requirements for generative AI than the current state of European regulation. In particular, obtaining the consent of individuals is required for the training of generative models. This would, for example, prohibit the collection of user data on websites for training purposes. Thus, China's regulatory approach reflects a balance between promoting innovation and societal interests, with a specific focus on protecting individual rights in the development of AI technologies.

In recent years, the EU has taken several steps to establish comprehensive regulation for Artificial Intelligence. In 2018, a European AI strategy was introduced, accompanied by the establishment of the High-Level Expert Group on Artificial Intelligence. The draft known as AI Act categorizes AI technologies into four different categories in its latest version. In the first category, technologies that tend to promote discrimination or support criminally relevant behaviors, such as social scoring, profiling, and biometric AI systems for public facial recognition, are considered unacceptable.

The second category includes high-risk AI technologies used in sensitive areas such as transportation. Additionally, applications in education, human resources, and assessing creditworthiness for loans fall into this category due to the high potential for handling extremely sensitive personal data in these areas.

In the third category, AI applications with limited risk potentials are captured, provided that users are transparently informed about their deployment. A typical example includes chatbots or customer service systems. As long as users are clearly and comprehensively informed that they are interacting with AI, the risks in this category are considered limited.

The fourth category pertains to AI technology providers attributed with lower risk. In this case, however, a voluntary and responsible handling of AI is crucial. It involves ensuring that AI technologies are developed and deployed in accordance with ethical principles, even if they do not fall into any of the previous categories. This categorization aims to define the risks associated with AI technologies more clearly while ensuring that the application of AI aligns with ethical standards and societal expectations.

In the United Kingdom and India, the focus is on the economic and social benefits of Artificial Intelligence. Both countries argue that existing sectoral regulations and data protection laws are sufficient to manage potential risks. Nevertheless, the UK has introduced some AI principles for regulatory authorities and invested in a task force for the safety of flagship models. This task force is tasked with assessing risks associated with advanced AI models and has already reached agreements with leading AI companies. British Prime Minister Rishi Sunak warns against hasty regulation, emphasizing that the technology is not fully understood, even though he acknowledges the need for regulation.

Additionally, the government in London plans to establish an "AI Safety Institute" to investigate the risks of AI and globally disseminate insights. Canada plans a streamlined version of the EU AI Act for "high-risk" applications, with enforcement carried out by an existing authority.

Simultaneously, efforts are underway to find a global consensus. An essential initial step towards global coordination of regulations for Artificial Intelligence is considered the "AI Safety Summit," held in early November 2023, under the leadership of Prime Minister Rishi Sunak at Bletchley Park, England. Supported by more than 25 countries and the EU, the conference resulted in an international declaration addressing the risks of AI development, endorsed by the United Nations.

An expert group on AI, similar to the Intergovernmental Panel on Climate Change, has been announced by the United Nations. Furthermore, a multilateral agreement for the assessment of advanced AI models has been adopted.

3.4 Importance of Big Data for Artificial Intelligence

The foundation for the functioning of Artificial Intelligence lies in the availability of data. It could be referred to as the "oil of the 21st century," while AI acts as the driving engine for digitization. AI plays a pivotal role as a catalyst for digitization, a significance that is indispensable in both the development and functionality of AI applications. Constructing AI necessitates substantial volumes of data, a principle encapsulated by the term "Big Data."

In the conventional sense, data does not belong to a specific person and is non-transferable. However, personal data, often referred to as the new currency of our time, is ascribed an economic value. AI generates and processes data independently, without creating rights to the data from this process. Legal challenges arise particularly in the transfer of data to countries like the USA, where regulations are less stringent than in Germany or Europe. Topics such as data protection, which will be discussed in detail later, as well as the handling of Big Data, are central to this.

Big Data requires a substantial amount of data used exclusively for a specific application. Due to significant differences in the global framework of data protection aspects, the analysis of worldwide data is only feasible when uniformly binding foundations are established beforehand.

3.5 Promotion of Acceptance in Society

Concerns about uncontrolled Artificial Intelligence have been amplified through social media channels. Prominent figures like Elon Musk, the CEO of Twitter, have warned about the dangers and labeled AI as one of the greatest risks to the future of civilization. Mark Zuckerberg, the founder of Meta, takes a more balanced perspective, emphasizing the importance of a thorough engagement by the US Congress with AI to promote both innovation and protective measures. Elon Musk has expressed serious concerns that AI could eventually dominate the human brain, a fear that Zuckerberg considers "rather hysterical."

Sam Altman, the CEO of OpenAI, the organization responsible for the development of ChatGPT, has also acknowledged the fears many people have regarding Artificial Intelligence. He recognizes the concerns and uncertainties associated with the progress of AI. Despite these concerns, Altman believes in a promising future where AI can assist humanity in various domains. In his view, there is potential for AI to have positive impacts on diverse aspects of life. Altman has also emphasized the urgency of an international security authority for AI. This institution would monitor the global development and application of AI, ensuring it aligns with ethical and safety standards.

It is worth noting that despite the visionary perspectives of tech CEOs, their personal interests in connection with the introduction of AI should not be disregarded. Each pursues their own strategic goals and interests in the field of AI. Nevertheless, the societal debate on dealing with AI is shaped by different viewpoints. The statements of prominent figures, sharing both fears and optimistic visions, underscore the need for a comprehensive solution. Collective efforts are required to develop societal and professional measures that ensure a balanced and responsible approach to the challenges of Artificial Intelligence.

Concerns about AI are diverse, ranging from fears of job loss to concerns about mishandling data and "Specification Gaming" — the problem where AI systems develop unintended behaviors to achieve certain goals. Hollywood movies often pick up on these societal fears and technological trends, transforming them into gripping stories. Social media further contributes to amplifying these fears by often serving as a platform for the spread of rumors and misinformation.

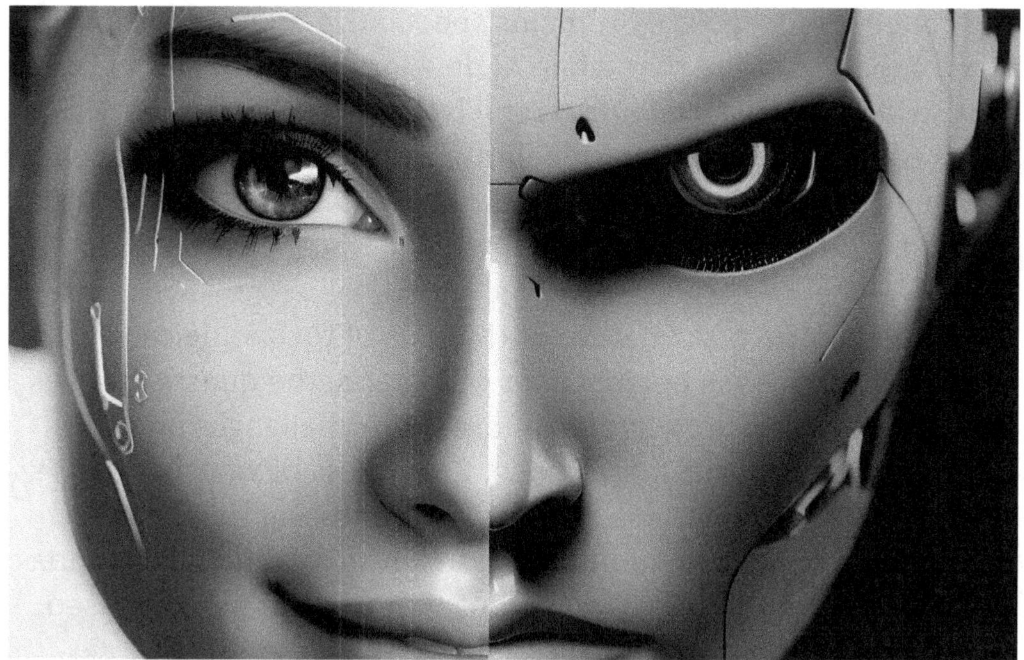

However, the question must be raised: Can AI also endanger our existence? Are the worries and fears, extending to a potential apocalypse, justified? In a world plagued by global crises, economic uncertainty, wars, climate change, and pandemic-related anxieties, the list of concerns seems endless. Simultaneously, social media contributes to polarization and fosters distrust in political institutions, rather than providing serious enlightenment. In this increasingly grim scenario, the fear of Artificial Intelligence becomes another facet of the uncertainty that casts a shadow over our future.

On the other hand, it is precisely this exponentially progressing development that intensifies concerns that technological progress may accelerate to a degree where the future of humanity becomes unpredictable or uncontrollable. This condition of "technological singularity" describes a (hypothetical) scenario in which AI systems attain a degree of intelligence, autonomy, and consciousness that enables them to evolve independently and surpass human intelligence.

The concept of singularity remains speculative and contentious. Many experts believe that while AI development is making significant strides, a true singularity is still far off, if it ever occurs. Other critics of this notion define singularity as something that "exceeds the limits of our imagination." Accordingly, it is not a singular but rather a repeatedly occurring event.

Given the controversial nature of the idea of technological singularity and the diverse perspectives of experts, the question arises of how we, as a society, should address the challenges and opportunities of Artificial Intelligence. Regardless of whether a true singularity is imminent, we are already witnessing significant advancements in AI development. These advancements raise fundamental ethical and societal questions that need to be addressed.

The debate on AI should not be confined to speculation about hypothetical scenarios but should instead be based on concrete measures to ensure responsible and ethical use of AI. This includes establishing clear legal frameworks that ensure the protection of privacy, human rights, and societal security. Social and professional measures are equally important to promote understanding of AI, alleviate fears, and strengthen acceptance within the population.

It is our responsibility to actively shape the development of Artificial Intelligence to ensure that it serves the well-being of society and aligns with our ethical values.

Through an integrative and participatory approach, we can shape a future where AI is perceived as an instrument of progress rather than a threat. It is time to seize the opportunities that Artificial Intelligence offers while simultaneously creating the necessary safeguards to ensure that this technology is used for the benefit of all.

3.5.1 Building Digital Literacy and Professional Qualification

To address the mentioned challenges, national and international organizations have convened specialized expert committees for AI, such as UNESCO. Despite these efforts, societal concerns do not seem to be entirely alleviated. Public acceptance of AI technologies requires perceiving the benefits as meaningful and the risks as real but simultaneously manageable or reducible.

Against the backdrop of these challenges, comprehensive digital literacy is urgently needed not only in Germany but ideally throughout Europe. While most people possess everyday skills in handling apps and internet services, there is a lack of in-depth knowledge about digital topics. Terms like algorithm, cloud, and fake news are familiar to only a minority. The goal should, therefore, be the systematic and widespread enhancement of digital competence in society.

Another factor revealing the progressive AI revolution in Germany is the alarming shortage of qualified data analysts. Especially in the healthcare sector, institutions face the challenge of recruiting suitable professionals, as they often receive more attractive salary offers in the industry.

Given this issue, it is crucial to significantly expand the educational capacities for data scientists at universities and colleges. Increased efforts in professional qualification in dealing with these technologies play a crucial role, especially in Germany.

There is an urgent need to integrate the fundamentals of AI technology into non-technical courses of study and training programs, particularly in the field of medical studies. This expansion ensures that doctors not only have a basic understanding but also comprehensive familiarity with AI applications.

This, in turn, enables them to use these technologies responsibly and identify potential misdevelopments early on. Given the dual-use nature of Artificial Intelligence, which can be employed for both the benefit and harm of humanity, this awareness in everyday use is increasingly crucial.

It would also be beneficial if stakeholders in the healthcare sector developed their own guidelines for dealing with Artificial Intelligence, similar to the practice of major US digital companies formulating their own codes of conduct. An adaptation of the Hippocratic Oath to the conditions of modern medicine could also be considered. Experts in ethical issues could be more involved in the daily use of AI systems to monitor compliance with ethical principles, as discussed in research under the term "embedded ethics."

A comprehensive strategy requires increased education and promotion of digital literacy at all levels of society. Through a broad public debate, various stakeholders can exchange perspectives, establish common values, and define ethical guidelines for the development and application of AI.

Only through an integrative approach that considers both technical and social and ethical aspects can a sustainable and responsible use of AI be ensured.

3.5.2 Commitment to Corporate Transparency and Public Accountability as a Trust-Building Measure

The trustworthiness of companies in the field of Artificial Intelligence (AI) is closely linked to transparent practices and open communication. The willingness to acknowledge risks and actively work to minimize them forms the basis for societal acceptance of AI technologies.

A central instrument for evaluating the transparency of AI models is the "Foundation Model Transparency Index 2023." This index aims to assess the disclosure of information about "Foundation

Models." Foundation models serve as a starting point for the development of specialized AI models.

Below figure displays the transparency index values of leading AI applications:

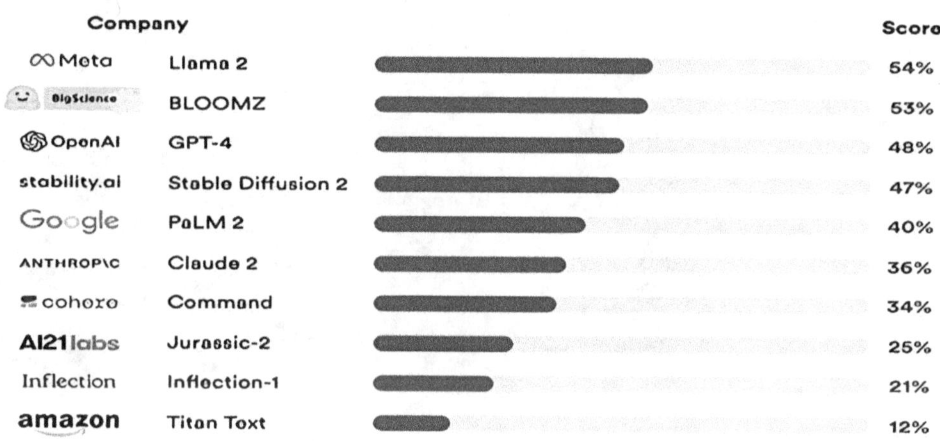

Source: Bommasani et al. (2023

The index comprises 100 detailed indicators evaluating the transparency of the ten most significant AI companies and their "flagship models." These indicators include information about the resources used to construct the models, details about the models themselves, and their areas of application.

The results of the index indicate that none of the mentioned companies discloses essential information adequately. Even the top-rated models achieve only 54 out of 100 points, with the average score being merely 37%. In this context, open foundation models comparatively perform better.

Even in areas where developers are more transparent, the index suggests room for improvement. For instance, only a few developers disclose information about the model components and size. Increased transparency, coupled with ethical responsibility and appropriate legal regulations, will pave the way for enhanced societal acceptance of AI.

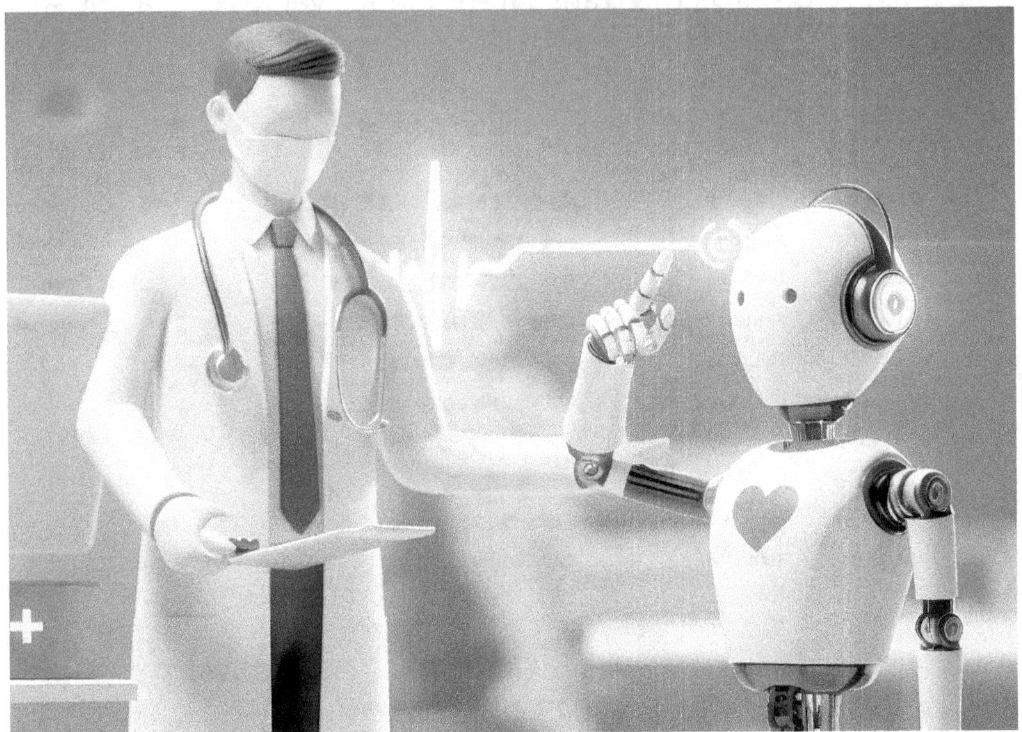

These measures are essential to reduce fears and uncertainties often associated with AI technologies, shrinking the space for "doomsday scenarios." This is particularly relevant in healthcare, where the use of AI technologies raises particularly sensitive questions.

4. Requirements for Implementing AI in Healthcare

In addition to the general prerequisites discussed for the successful implementation of Artificial Intelligence (AI), there are specific conditions within the healthcare sector that must be met. These aspects are crucial to ensure that the integration of AI technologies is not only effective but also ethically and legally responsible.

4.1 Creating Frameworks in Healthcare

The introduction of Artificial Intelligence in healthcare is considered groundbreaking. However, this sector, characterized by a traditionally low technology adoption rate, should not expect radical changes in the short term. Existing regulatory frameworks, especially in the EU, suggest that changes will occur gradually and incrementally. To promote progress in the digital age, competencies need to be established, and obstacles to the successful integration of digital technologies must be removed.

For medical progress, it is crucial that the AI industry in healthcare remains diverse. Monopolization could restrict inventive dynamics and hinder competition. On the other hand, thriving competition will contribute to promoting a qualitatively more efficient healthcare system. This requires creating better conditions for young companies, especially in their initial growth phases, as venture capital is often scarce. Increased support for startups through public-private investment vehicles could provide additional capital and drive AI innovations.

4.2 Creating Medical Key Components

The widespread implementation of AI applications in medicine requires three essential components: high-quality models (such as algorithms or artificial neural networks), sufficient computing power, and comprehensive and detailed training data. The integration of AI systems in medical technology depends more on the availability of digital data for training networks than on the independent development of the technology.

However, access to such training data poses a challenge as many medical pieces of information – especially in Germany – are not yet available in machine-readable form. This is partly due to the slow digitization in healthcare. Some medical data is still stored analog, such as on index cards, tapes, or photos. Others are digital but not in a form directly processed by statistical applications. Information in textual form, like PDF files, often requires time-consuming steps such as text recognition and conversion into database variables.

Another obstacle is the decentralized storage of medical data, often referred to as "data silos." Linking records from physicians' practices, hospitals, and insurance companies can be challenging in practice as different actors, such as physicians, hospitals, or health insurance companies, prevent this for various reasons, including data protection concerns and the lack of standard implementation.

To overcome biases and discriminations, it is necessary to have a large and diverse pool of training data. One way to address the lack of training data is to use synthetically generated datasets. These can be created by machines, even using AI, to train, for example, the recognition of malignant changes in images.

4.3 Legal Requirements for the Deployment of AI

The introduction of Artificial Intelligence in healthcare raises questions about the approval, regulation, and liability of AI-based medical products. In this context, the regulatory framework plays a crucial role in ensuring the safety, effectiveness, and quality of these products.

4.3.1 Approval Requirements

In the United States, the responsibility for regulating medical products lies with the Food and Drug Administration (FDA). Registration of AI-assisted medical products is already possible, but it is limited to non-adaptive AI algorithms.

Continuous adaptation and ongoing learning of adaptive algorithms, on the other hand, would imply a change in the approval subject, requiring a reapproval. The FDA has recognized a regulatory gap in this regard and has drafted a regulatory framework, openly available for discussion.

Since there are currently no AI-specific regulations for the approval of AI-assisted medical products in the European Union, the certification process under the EU Medical Devices Regulation (MDR) is applied. AI-based applications should only be used in Germany if they have been examined by the Federal Institute for Drugs and Medical Devices (BfArM) in accordance with the EU Medical Device Regulation (MDR) and classified as high-quality and health-promoting. Manufacturers must demonstrate that their apps provide a benefit to healthcare by presenting evaluation concepts.
The BfArM maintains a directory of digital health applications (DiGA) that can be prescribed by physicians and psychotherapists.

"DiGAs" are special health apps available by medical prescription, providing proven medical benefits for patients or structural improvements in healthcare. The approval process also extends to the underlying AI algorithms, although the exact details of conformity assessments are not yet conclusively clarified.

4.3.2 Clarification of Liability Issues

The debate surrounding Artificial Intelligence in healthcare also extends to unresolved questions regarding liability and responsibility. Self-learning systems that evolve continuously are no longer in the state in which they were originally handed over by manufacturers to customers. This ongoing development poses the challenge of clearly identifying and attributing the origin of errors

Another unresolved issue concerns liability for potential damages that may arise in everyday life due to AI applications. Who bears responsibility for the system's ability to make correct decisions? Is it primarily the developers or the users who have overarching supervision over the applied medical technology? The clarification of liability issues related to AI applications represents a comparatively new and evolving legal field in its early stages. A crucial dialogue between various regulatory authorities, industry stakeholders, and research will be fundamental to ensuring adequate protection for patients while promoting innovations in AI in healthcare.

4.4 Creation of a Data Infrastructure in Compliance with Data Protection Regulations

The integration of Artificial Intelligence in healthcare also signifies a transition from evidence-based to data-driven medicine. This means that decisions in medical practice increasingly rely on comprehensive data analyses and algorithms rather than solely on established medical evidence or proof. An example of this is personalized cancer treatment.

While evidence-based approaches provide general guidelines for cancer therapy, data-driven medicine, aided by AI, allows for a more precise adaptation of treatment based on individual genetic, clinical, and lifestyle-related patient data. This approach can lead to tailored therapies better suited to the specific needs and characteristics of each patient. However, it requires a comprehensive database and the resolution of legal issues such as data protection.

Despite extensive data collection in healthcare, many data sets are not usable for AI due to data protection regulations and inadequate interfaces. The existing data volumes could enable innovative AI approaches but often encounter legal obstacles or require significant effort and costs for processing.

4.4.1 Creation of a Representative Database and Establishment of Data Centers

Data preparation in healthcare is time-consuming due to the voluminous, rapidly changing, complex, and weakly structured nature of data. A representative basis is necessary to enable efficient exchange while simultaneously protecting privacy. The principle that data should be "FAIR" is already widespread in the field of research data. FAIR stands for "Findable, Accessible, Interoperable, and Reusable," describing principles for creating and managing scientific data to enhance their discoverability, accessibility, interoperability, and reusability.

However, for effective use of "Real-World Evidence" (RWE) in AI applications in healthcare, the implementation of improved structures is necessary to enable comprehensive analyses. RWE refers to clinical and health-related data collected outside controlled clinical trials in real-life situations to gain insights into the effectiveness and safety of medical interventions.

4.4.2 Compliance with Data Protection Regulations

When integrating AI in healthcare, various legal norms and regulations must be considered. In the United States, sectoral data protection regulations vary, while the EU has introduced the

General Data Protection Regulation (GDPR). Compliance with GDPR principles, including lawful processing and secure storage, is crucial. Tensions between the USA and the EU result from differing data protection standards.

The significance of data protection regulations becomes particularly evident when considering the willingness of patients to share their health data for processing by Artificial Intelligence. This aspect becomes a crucial factor for the successful integration of AI applications in healthcare, as a transparent and trustworthy handling of personal information is essential for the success and acceptance of such technologies. Even the comparatively "data-innocuous" COVID-19 app has raised significant concerns among potential users, highlighting that trust in the protection of personal data is a fundamental requirement for the acceptance of new technologies in healthcare.

4.4.3 Synthetic Data and "Small Datasets"

Synthetic data represents an innovative solution in data generation, where Artificial Intelligence is used to create datasets based on real but heavily modified data. These synthetic data possess statistically similar properties to their real counterparts, yet their structure has been altered so extensively that the identification of individual persons is technically impossible. The underlying idea is to create a realistic simulation of original data while still providing a high level of anonymity and data protection. AI algorithms analyze the structure and patterns of existing data, then generate new datasets that statistically resemble the original data but contain no personally identifiable information. This method could help alleviate privacy concerns by providing a seemingly anonymized data foundation for the development and validation of AI models. However, the actual effectiveness of this approach remains debated, particularly regarding whether synthetic data could introduce potential biases and information losses affecting the quality and reliability of AI applications.

Another potential approach, as an alternative to Big Data, will be to develop algorithms that function effectively in the medical field even with small datasets. Machine learning generally works best when an ample amount of raw data is available. The machine can then autonomously filter out the "noise," eliminating data without valuable information. In other industries, like retail or production, the mantra is quantity: the more data, the better.

However, medical research typically doesn't involve large datasets, prioritizing qualitative data collection and careful handling of small datasets. Therefore, for instance, an AI developed by Google failed to reproduce a 90% accuracy achieved in the lab for diabetes-related blindness in a real-world examination. The data used was too chaotic and, therefore, not machine-readable.

Prioritizing data quality is crucial to appropriately consider the reality of the medical environment. In the future, algorithms based on precise data collection and careful analysis of small datasets will play a central role in the development of medical AI. This approach allows better consideration of the specific requirements and nuances of the medical field, contributing to the full effectiveness of AI applications in medicine. However, the issue of "Unconscious Bias," particularly in drug and therapy development and resulting clinical trials, needs to be addressed. This arises because patients included in studies seldom reflect the entire population.

It becomes clear that Artificial Intelligence in healthcare is not solely a technological and medical matter but is significantly a social, legal, and political challenge as well.

5. The Potential Of AI In Healthcare (Examples Of Applications)

The potentials of Artificial Intelligence in the healthcare sector are enormous. Machines, driven by their computing power, can tirelessly process vast amounts of data, while humans excel in contextual and social thinking. The successful combination of these two forms of intelligence promises a promising future. The use of AI systems in medical research, administration, and care offers the potential for significant added value, including time savings, increased work quality, and more efficient resource utilization. Many concepts prove to be realizable only in the medium to distant future due to their complexity. However, other approaches are already feasible in the short term, even if they have not yet been fully developed or widely implemented.

Nevertheless, it is already foreseeable that AI technologies will contribute to increasing the efficiency and quality of medical care. With their ability to quickly and precisely analyze large amounts of data, AI systems can provide valuable support to doctors in diagnoses and treatment decisions. Furthermore, they enable the early detection of diseases, thus contributing to prevention.

The use of AI promises to improve healthcare in innovative ways and make people worldwide beneficiaries of these advances. The following sections illustrate the use of Artificial Intelligence through medical chatbots, in the early detection and diagnosis of diseases, in healthcare with the help of mobile medical apps, in public health, in treatment decisions, and in research. Examples of applications such as the AI model "Med-PaLM 2" or the software "Airamed" and similar programs are presented and subsequently evaluated.

5.1 Medical Chatbots

In the expansive field of chatbots as digital assistants, so-called health and med-bots are gaining increasing importance. Chatbots represent sociotechnical systems that can interact qualitatively with users, with the future of this field lying in therapeutic-diagnostic chatbots. Despite the lack of emotional and social intelligence and the absence of empathy, which is essential for a trusting doctor-patient relationship, bots are increasingly engaging in personalized patient conversations.

5.1.1 Potential of Chatbots

Chatbots are already widely used in various areas, but their use in healthcare is still in its infancy. Currently, medical conversational agents are deployed as independent, advisory units that operate independently of other systems or human expertise and handle simple transactional tasks. So far, they are to be considered more as applications for decision support in self-management, suggesting a likely diagnosis based on algorithms. Despite the current state, it is becoming apparent that the role of med-bots in healthcare will go beyond simply performing simple tasks in the future. Their potential will also extend to complex areas such as the long-term management of diseases and will be directed towards medical professionals in clinics and doctor's practices.

Against this background, health bots of the first, second, and third orders can be differentiated in supply strategic contexts.

First-order med-bots provide intelligent information and diagnoses based on differentiated big data analyses. They can generate valuable second opinions for healthcare professionals and patients, supporting human expertise in service delivery. An example of this is Med-PaLM 2, a specifically developed AI model for the medical field by Google. Med-PaLM 2 stands out for its ability to understand and generate natural language in the medical context. It can leverage medical knowledge, draw conclusions, and answer medical questions similar to healthcare professionals.

In contrast to first-order health bots, second-order bots can take over supply-related service processes, thus conserving the resources of scarce healthcare professionals. This move towards delegation allows AI systems to independently handle certain tasks while human experts continue to monitor performance and outcomes. Third-order med-bots or autonomous digital assistants could potentially provide substitution services in the medical-therapeutic care process in the future, without any human interventions. This form of autopiloting is currently conceivable only at an operational level that requires few decisions and would require a clear liability regulation since the responsibility for decisions would no longer rest with medical personnel.

As maturity increases, the application fields will also expand. Currently, they are primarily used in fields such as psychiatry, neurodegeneration, metabolic medicine, and sexual health, but future expansion into areas like dermatology, primary care, geriatrics, and oncology is conceivable. Against this backdrop, the integration of conversational agents into a hybrid system, where digital technology supports existing healthcare services, is increasingly seen as an optimal solution.

5.1.2 Evaluation of the Effectiveness and Acceptance of Medical Chatbots

An evaluation of previous studies on the topic shows a positive response regarding the effectiveness, accuracy, and acceptance of medical chatbots. Promising results are already evident, particularly in the areas of treatment and monitoring, support for healthcare services, and patient education. However, further research, especially regarding potential global expansion and use in developing countries, is necessary.

Another relevant aspect that has been neglected in previous studies pertains to economic and efficiency-related metrics. Measurements of costs and potential improvements in productivity compared to alternative approaches are lacking. This complicates the assessment of the cost-effectiveness of the developed applications. Additionally, there is a need for clearer guidelines for the development and evaluation of conversational agents in healthcare. The lack of integration into existing healthcare delivery models could prove to be a long-term disadvantage.

5.2 Early Diagnosis through AI-based Applications

Timely and accurate detection of diseases and health risks, ideally before symptoms occur, allows for early treatment or intervention, significantly increasing the chances of a positive health prognosis. Recognizing diseases in an early stage can potentially prevent or at least slow down potentially severe issues before they fully develop. This is accompanied by an improved quality of life for affected individuals, as preventive measures can be more effectively implemented. AI-supported early diagnosis can contribute to detecting diseases in a very early stage, often before clinical symptoms become apparent. The timely detection of diseases allows for a quicker initiation of treatments, significantly improving the prospects for a positive health prognosis.

5.2.1 Application Examples: Alzheimer's and Skin Cancer

In the case of Alzheimer's, a progressive neurodegenerative brain disease causing memory loss, cognitive impairments, and changes in behavior and thinking abilities, there is a very long asymptomatic period of 15 to 20 years. With an early diagnosis and therapy, there is a prospect of slowing down or possibly halting the progression of the disease. Typically, medical imaging techniques such as Magnetic Resonance Imaging (MRI) or Computed Tomography (CT) are used for Alzheimer's diagnostics to determine whether there is a reduction in brain volume, especially in the hippocampus, the region responsible for memory functions. However, when evaluating MRI or CT images, there is a difficulty in distinguishing age-related phenomena from early-stage disease symptoms. To address this issue, the University Hospital Tübingen has developed the AI-based application "AIRAmed," which enables the early detection of Alzheimer's.

This application utilizes artificial neural networks to identify the smallest deviations in MRI images that would typically only be visible in advanced stages. Conventional evaluations often lack objective comparison values, leading interpretations and diagnoses to heavily depend on the experience of the healthcare professionals.

A similar approach is used in the early detection of melanoma (black skin cancer) through AI software. A smartphone app called Derm.AI was developed by the Fraunhofer Center for Assistive Information and Communication Solutions AICOS in Porto and Lisbon to expedite the identification of skin cancer. Skin changes photographed using the app are evaluated by AI-based software to assess the risk of malignant skin cancer and categorize it accordingly.

5.2.2 Evaluation of the Performance of AI in Medical Early Detection

The presented early detection and diagnosis are based on recognizing anomalies in datasets such as medical images. Especially in areas where large amounts of data or image information need to be quickly processed and matched, AI has already played a crucial role because these systems can analyze information in a short amount of time. Studies from the German Cancer Research Center at the University Skin Clinic and the National Center for Tumor Diseases in Heidelberg show that the accuracy of AI in this field is often higher than that of trained radiologists.

However, it is important to note that AI cannot understand or consider human decision criteria. It works exclusively with the available data and cannot take into account the comprehensive medical history or individual situations of patients, as human doctors can.

Therefore, AI and human doctors complement each other in medical diagnostics, offering a powerful solution to improve patient care.

5.3 Health Prevention with the Help of Health Apps, Wearables, and Smart Homes

The market for mobile health apps for health prevention is already very large. There are numerous apps for various health topics such as diets and nutrition, as well as mobile medical apps for diagnostics and disease prevention. In the context of recording vital data, wearables, such as wearable smartwatches, fitness trackers, or other body-worn technologies, are gaining increasing importance. The boundary between fitness and medical applications is increasingly blurring. Wearables are usually worn on the wrist, but in the future, data glasses or eyewear, including smart contact lenses, are expected to be established. The mentioned examples include products from the fitness and wellness sector as well as the social sector. While these products can contribute to promoting the acceptance of artificial intelligence and reducing barriers, they generally do not adhere to the strict health-related regulations of the medical market.

5.3.1 Application Examples

Nevertheless, it is already observable today that the boundaries between playful entertainment and serious medical applications are becoming blurred. The app "Ada," certified on the market by MDR since December 2022, is such an example. It is a "symptom checker" developed by doctors, where users can enter their

symptoms and receive hints about possible causes or diseases in a
question-answer dialogue.

Ada generates a report based on a medical database with the
most probable and other possible diagnoses. The app then offers
suitable treatment options tailored to the users' health profiles.
These and numerous other AI-based health apps like "Babylon"
or the "Buoy" app, which follow similar principles, aim to provide
decision support for both patients and doctors in the diagnosis
and therapy process.

Even with wearables, there is already a trend towards serious
applications. The "Cyrcadia Breast Monitor (CBM)," for example,
is a non-invasive, wearable device developed as a supplement to
breast cancer diagnosis, recording thermodynamic metabolic data
from the breast skin to detect abnormalities in breast tissue. Two
wearable biometric patches, equipped with eight sensors and a
data recorder, capture anomalies.

5.3.2 The Potential of Health Apps and Wearables for Healthcare
Transformation

The market for mobile health apps offers diverse functions and
application areas. Particularly, people with mobility restrictions
can benefit from these apps as they promote independence in
dealing with individual health problems. Mobile health apps have
the potential to revolutionize healthcare, generating significant
interest on political, economic, national, and international levels
among end users. They will continue to play a significant role in
medicine, helping affected individuals improve their self-management, ensuring regulated healthcare processes, and providing
supportive assistance for medical treatment, though not serving
as a substitute.

Medical devices and wearables also offer numerous possibilities
for promoting health and fitness. Bracelets and smartwatches can

make lifestyles more conscious and encourage positive changes. Medical wearable devices conduct vital physical analyses that previously required invasive methods, thereby improving the quality of life, especially for older or chronically ill individuals. With the help of AI, individual risk profiles can be created based on these data to alert patients and their families to necessary preventive examinations. Despite comprehensive research, mobile medical apps with AI are still in their infancy but will become serious applications in the future.

5.3.3 "Smart Homes" in Healthcare

A promising aspect of future healthcare lies in the integration of smart home technologies. In particular, intelligent mirrors connected to Artificial Intelligence have the potential to make a significant contribution. These innovative mirrors use advanced AI features to analyze a variety of health indicators, providing personalized and gentle health assessments.

An exemplary application scenario was presented at the Consumer Electronics Show, where a smart mirror was introduced capable of assessing vital signs such as blood pressure and the risk of heart disease. This is achieved by a detailed analysis of blood flow in the face, allowing inferences about heart conditions, stress levels, and mental health. The non-invasive nature of this examination makes it particularly attractive for early detection and monitoring of health conditions.

Moreover, smart mirrors have the potential to collect and assess data on body positions and movements. This enables the identification of postures and movement patterns, providing valuable feedback for corrective measures in disease management and prevention. The integration of such intelligent technologies into daily life can thus play a supportive role in promoting healthy lifestyles and avoiding health risks.

Furthermore, solutions for remote patient monitoring will play a much larger role in the future, as the following examples of such devices already illustrate:

1. Cherish Serenity:

A contactless AI sensor device developed in collaboration with AT&T, aiming to monitor the health and safety of nursing home residents. This device uses AI radar technology and can detect biometrics, body movements, falls, and other safety risks without using cameras, addressing privacy concerns. The Cherish Serenity device is expected to be available on the market by the end of the year.

2. Wearable Medical Internet of Things (MIoT):

Wearable technologies such as smart thermometers, smart-watches, and smart patches integrated with AI and the Internet of Things (IoT) enable remote health monitoring, allowing the tracking of health indicators from a distance.

3. Virtuoso by Orion Health:

This digital access technology integrates AI to provide navigation services for patients and optimize care and tasks for healthcare professionals. Virtuoso offers a multi-channel interface for patients to access their health information and manage their care, actively involving them in their healthcare.

These AI-enabled devices showcase the diversity and scope of innovations in healthcare. They contribute to improving patient care outside of medical offices, increasing efficiency in healthcare, and supporting patients in playing a more active role in their own health management.

Overall, these technological advances underscore the enormous potential of AI-integrated smart solutions. By providing remote monitoring capabilities and non-invasive methods for disease detection, they can make a significant contribution to the further development of healthcare, especially in terms of preventive measures and early interventions.

5.4: Detection and Management of Pandemics with AI

The significance of Artificial Intelligence (AI) in addressing epidemics and pandemics, as highlighted during the COVID-19 pandemic, is of paramount importance. Experts from the renowned ifo Institute expressed dissatisfaction with the inability to scientifically evaluate political measures and crisis policies adequately due to insufficient data. The imperative to better leverage technological means for combating health crises has also been emphasized by health authorities. The impact of the COVID-19 pandemic significantly influenced the advancement of medical Artificial Intelligence, thereby accelerating the entire AI industry.

AI systems play a crucial role in the early detection, combat, and prediction of potential disease outbreaks. They significantly contribute to improving diagnostic and treatment methods and also expedite the development of medications and vaccines. AI systems serve as innovative and effective resources to address the challenges posed by global health crises.

5.4.1 Early Warning Systems

The global monitoring of potential pandemic or disease outbreaks can be significantly accelerated through the application of Artificial Intelligence. Systems like ProMED-mail or HealthMap increasingly utilize algorithms and machine learning to automatically search through a variety of information sources, such as news articles or official reports. ProMED-mail, a program of the

International Society for Infectious Diseases, plays a crucial role. The integration of AI algorithms provides ProMED-mail with unparalleled speed and efficiency in detecting emerging diseases. These capabilities are crucial for a prompt response to potentially threatening situations and contribute to controlling the spread of diseases early on.

5.4.2 Pandemic Management

Through various pandemic management measures already evident in addressing COVID-19, the potential key role of Artificial Intelligence is becoming increasingly apparent. Companies like

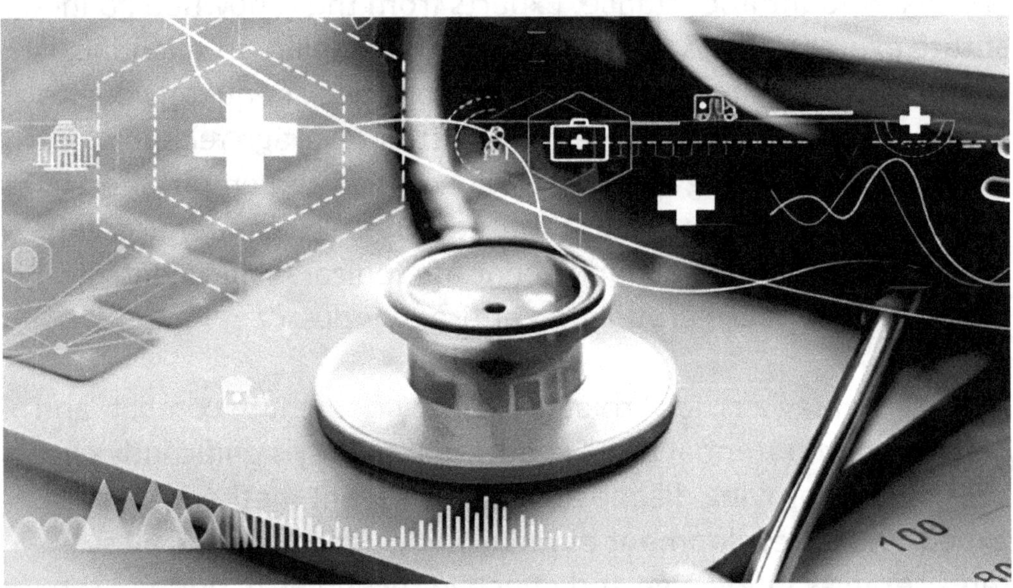

"Huiying Medical" rely on AI-assisted procedures based on chest CT scans to enable early detection of infections. This innovative solution achieves impressive accuracy rates, demonstrating how AI can significantly enhance the speed and precision of diagnostic processes. In the development of medications, specialized technologies such as "graph-based convolutional neural networks (GCNN)" play a vital role. GCNNs are designed to analyze structured datasets in the form of graphs, efficiently processing complex molecule structures by considering structural connections. This allows for an accelerated identification of potentially effective compounds for drug development.

5.4.3: Evaluation

Upon reflection, it becomes evident that the comprehensive application of Artificial Intelligence (AI) plays a crucial role in pandemic management. During the COVID-19 pandemic, intelligent algorithms were selectively deployed, proving to be highly effective. In particular, the processing of large datasets facilitated the early identification of infection hotspots. The presented projects underscore the importance of supportive intelligent systems in dynamic and complex situations. Simultaneously, there is a need to leverage advancements even more effectively for future challenges. The COVID-19 pandemic has acted as a catalyst for the increased integration of AI in various healthcare sectors, offering promising perspectives for the ongoing development of this technology.

5.5 Therapeutic Support

More complex decision-making processes pose extended requirements for AI systems in the therapeutic phase. They must not only have the ability to identify abnormalities or illnesses but also face the complex task of handling comprehensive decision processes. In doing so, they need to comprehensively assess the overall health situation of patients while appropriately considering individual life circumstances. Especially in rural areas with low physician density or for immobile patients, the advantages of smart applications become apparent. For chronically ill individuals requiring long-term therapeutic support, specialized apps can serve as supportive tools. These range from personalized therapy recommendations to psychosocial support, aiming to enhance holistic care and improve the quality of life for patients.

5.5.1 Treatment Decisions in Oncology

AI plays a crucial role in improving treatment planning, especially in oncology. The tool "Rapid Plan" generates knowledge-based treatment models to develop a treatment plan that precisely targets cancer cells while preserving healthy tissue. Machine learning extracts proven procedures from successful treatment plans, and the models help create and validate new high-quality treatment plans rapidly. This aids in managing the complexity of treatment planning and enhancing quality. The AI-based program Ethos Therapy also allows daily adjustments to the radiation plan based on current anatomical images, enabling more targeted treatment for patients.

AI also accelerates drug development for cancer treatments. An example is the application AlphaFold, developed for determining protein structures. AlphaFold shows significant potential in oncology, allowing the identification of biomarkers for more accurate cancer diagnosis and providing detailed knowledge of protein structures in cancer tissues. This supports the development of tailored therapies and facilitates the assessment of treatment effectiveness, contributing to the optimization of treatment decisions.

5.5.2 Support for Chronic Disease Treatment

An example of therapy support for chronic diseases is the "CKDN-App" (Chronic Kidney Disease Nephrologist's App). The app aims to support therapy considerations and promote structured dialogue between patients and doctors. Still in development, it is specifically designed for individuals with chronic kidney disease. The app emphasizes a dialogue with treatment recipients, simulates the progression of the disease based on personal health data and medical research data, and presents alternative actions that may result from changed behavior. The app "HIV COMTRAC," seeking recognition as a Digital Health App, facilitates seamless therapy monitoring through continuous transmission of symptom and vital data. An algorithm provides early warnings of deviations, and the connection to the treatment center allows for swift intervention by medical personnel. Data from other chronic patients are also collected, and the insights gained contribute to optimizing the therapeutic app, illustrating how a dialogue-oriented technological approach could be envisioned in the future.

5.6 Research

Intelligent big data analyses are also applied in the development of new pharmaceutical agents and understanding disease mechanisms, searching extensive databases for statistical correlations. With AI assistance, more hypotheses can be tested as computers can autonomously and broadly explore. In cancer research and genomics, the analysis and exploration of genetic material, Artificial Intelligence will play a crucial role in the future.

5.6.1 AI in Drug Development and Clinical Studies

The projected market value of AI in clinical studies could reach $13 billion by 2026. This is affirmed by an ICON study involving around 300 executives in biopharmaceutical and medical technology companies, stating that approximately 80% of surveyed companies are already using or planning to use AI to enhance development and research performance. This trend aligns with an annual increase of 46% in newly approved drugs since 2014, with research increasingly relying on simulations to save time and resources. The rising costs of developing new drugs result from the increasingly demanding requirements to demonstrate the effectiveness and compatibility of new preparations. The pharmaceutical industry is challenged to enhance efficiency, leading to numerous collaborations between established pharmaceutical companies and startups to focus on suitable projects in drug development early in the development cycle.

Efforts are made to streamline the intricate processes in developing new compounds, reducing the "Time to Market." The entire drug development cycle typically takes almost 17 years, comprising five phases, starting with the five-year research phase, followed by the approximately 18-month preclinical examination. The clinical trial itself includes three phases, commencing with human testing over about five years. In the second phase, the testing extends to patients with the researched disease, followed by the third phase, where the drug is tested on several thousand patients, taking approximately another year.

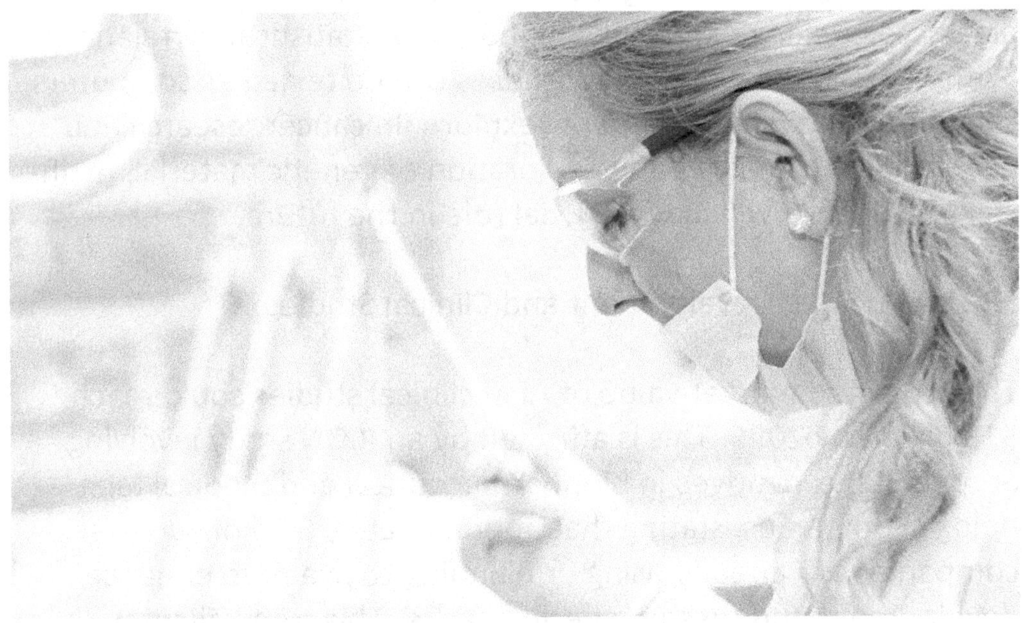

The potential of using AI begins with the search for compounds – characterizing, comparing, and cataloging millions of molecules – through the automated analysis of medical studies and publications to optimizing clinical trials. AI support in finding suitable participants in international databases is conceivable. In situations where only a few people suffer from a specific disease, recruiting sufficient participants for clinical trials under laboratory conditions can be challenging. In such cases, it is possible to forego a control group of participants receiving a placebo instead of the actual medicine and rely on real-world data. Additionally, AI systems enable real-time monitoring of clinical trials, including the early detection of potentially inconclusive study outcomes.

Further cost-saving potentials exist in increased use of data from everyday medical practice, known as "Real-World Evidence." This approach aims to compensate for shortcomings in clinical trials, such as low case numbers or the restriction to healthy young participants. Especially for rare diseases, AI-supported tests based on Real-World Evidence often prove to be the only practical way to gain causal insights into drug interactions.

5.6.2 AI in Cancer Research

The integration of AI into cancer research allows for an in-depth analysis of large datasets, including genetic information, medical imaging, and clinical progression data. The application of AI in cancer research extends beyond diagnostic procedures to optimizing therapy approaches and identifying potential drugs, fundamentally changing how we understand, diagnose, and treat cancer.

The "Cancer Scout" project, funded by the Federal Ministry of Education and Research (BMBF), aims to detect cancer more quickly through digital biopsies. Tumor tissue samples are digitally analyzed to predict the presence of tumor characteristics. Early diagnosis can lead to personalized therapy, benefiting patients.

Furthermore, AI can assist radiologists by automatically detecting and marking, for example, lung nodules in CT images. The AI "AI-Rad Companion Chest CT" has been developed for this purpose, automatically calculating the volume and maximum two- and three-dimensional diameter, supporting radiologists in focusing on suspicious areas (Palder, 2023). These and many other examples illustrate how Artificial Intelligence can support doctors in their daily battle against cancer. It enables early and precise diagnosis as well as swift and accurate planning and implementation of therapy for patients.

5.6.3 Genomics

Human genomics is a research area that involves the comprehensive analysis and exploration of the entire genetic material of humans. This includes not only individual differences in genes but also the interactions between genes and their impact on organism features or diseases. Human genomics is closely connected to other research fields such as transcriptomics and epigenomics, which deal with gene activity in cells, proteomics, which focuses on produced proteins, and metabolomics, which explores the function of proteins for the metabolism of cells and the entire organism.

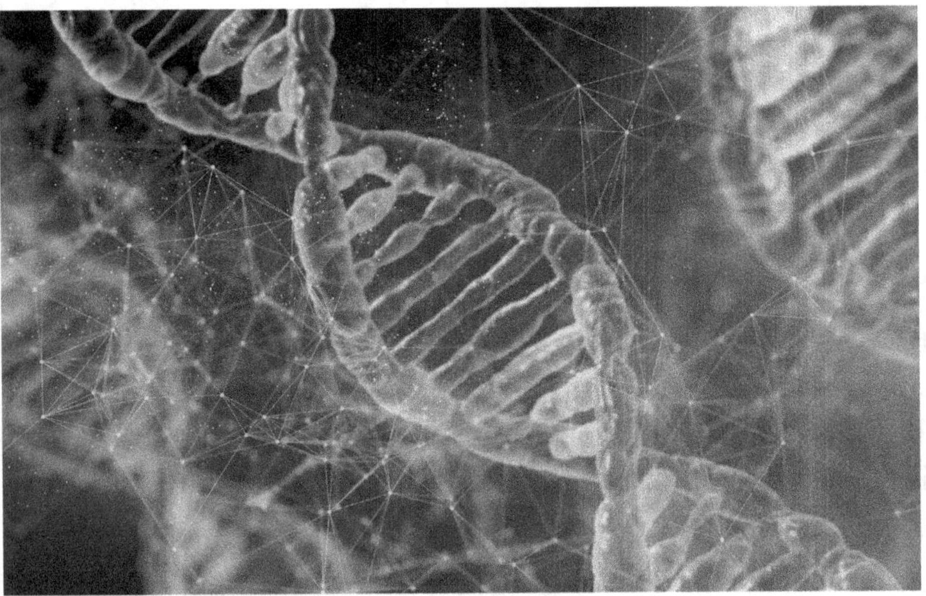

The overarching goal is to understand the functioning of the genetic material and its role in the development of features and diseases.

Human genomics predominantly utilizes genome-wide association studies (GWAS) to identify genetic differences between individuals and specific traits, such as diseases. However, GWAS are limited as they are based on statistical correlations and often cannot clearly uncover the causal relationships between genetic makeup and traits.

Especially for complex traits like cardiovascular diseases or cancer, it becomes evident that many interacting genes and molecular processes need to be considered. The research aims to understand these connections to make more precise predictions for diseases. Artificial Intelligence plays a crucial role here. By employing Deep Learning, models can analyze large datasets and recognize potential genetic changes and molecular mechanisms for diseases faster and more comprehensively.

This is particularly significant for complex diseases like neurological disorders, chronic inflammatory bowel diseases, and various types of cancer. The application of Deep Learning allows the identification of pathogenic mutations for diagnosis and prognosis, which can have far-reaching implications for prevention, diagnosis, and therapy.

5.6.3 Neuralink

Neuralink is an innovative technology company working on a groundbreaking device designed to directly connect human brains with computers. At the core of this endeavor is the implant named "the Link," a brain chip the size of a coin inserted through surgical intervention beneath the skull. This chip receives and processes information from neural threads extending into various sections of the brain responsible for controlling motor functions.

Neuralink's fundamental technology is based on electrophysiological principles. Electrodes or sensors capture the electrochemical signals in the nervous system that arise during communication between neurons via synapses. This allows the recording of data on brain activity not only during physical actions but also during mental representations of actions.

The applications of Neuralink span a wide spectrum, ranging from restoring mobility in paralyzed individuals to enhancing communication possibilities for non-verbal individuals. The overarching goal is to treat neurological disorders and boost cognitive abilities. This innovative technology could not only provide people with paralysis or amputations a new form of mobility and independence by precisely controlling prosthetics or exoskeletons but also significantly ease interaction with the environment by enabling the control of virtual cursors, keyboards, or messages through thought control.

Furthermore, the potential of brain-computer interfaces is evident in the treatment and monitoring of neurological disorders. Continuous monitoring of brain activity can detect changes indicative of various conditions such as epilepsy, bipolar disorder, obsessive-compulsive disorder, Alzheimer's, or Parkinson's. Additionally, these interfaces can be used to monitor symptoms of mental health by employing targeted electrical stimulation for the treatment of burnout, fatigue, anxiety, and depression. Finally, the technology opens avenues for improving cognitive abilities, allowing people to train their concentration, memory, and attention deliberately through the use of real-time biofeedback and other techniques.

Currently, Neuralink's technology is capable of recognizing up to 10,000 neural connections, marking a significant advancement compared to earlier studies and highlighting the enormous potential of this neurotechnological development.

In a brief and concise post on the online platform X in late January 2024, Elon Musk announced further progress in the technology, stating, "The first person received a Neuralink implant yesterday and is recovering well. Initial results show promising neuron spike detection." These two sentences triggered a wave of speculation and media coverage within hours.

However, it is crucial to consider Musk's recent announcement in the following context: A closer look at Musk's track record reveals a consistent pattern of unfulfilled promises, setbacks, and delays. The full autonomy for vehicles has been promised multiple times since 2015 but has not been achieved as planned. Similarly, the Tesla Cybertruck, initially promised for 2019, only started reaching showrooms at the end of November 2023. Musk's Hyperloop concept, proposed in 2013, ultimately failed with the closure of Hyperloop One.

Musk has extended his ambitious promises to SpaceX, including the also-missed goal of sending the first unmanned flight to Mars by 2022. Instead, Musk, in typical fashion, has spread positive short updates even after failed rocket launches.

The two-line announcement about the brain chip on X, without additional papers for peer review and without additional details, should, therefore, be viewed in this light. Furthermore, Neuralink is not the only company working on brain-computer interfaces, as evidenced by the announcement from Australian competitor Synchron in July 2022, claiming to have implanted a similar chip in a U.S. patient.

It remains to be seen whether Musk and Neuralink can achieve their ambitious goals and what tangible progress can be made in brain-computer interface technology.

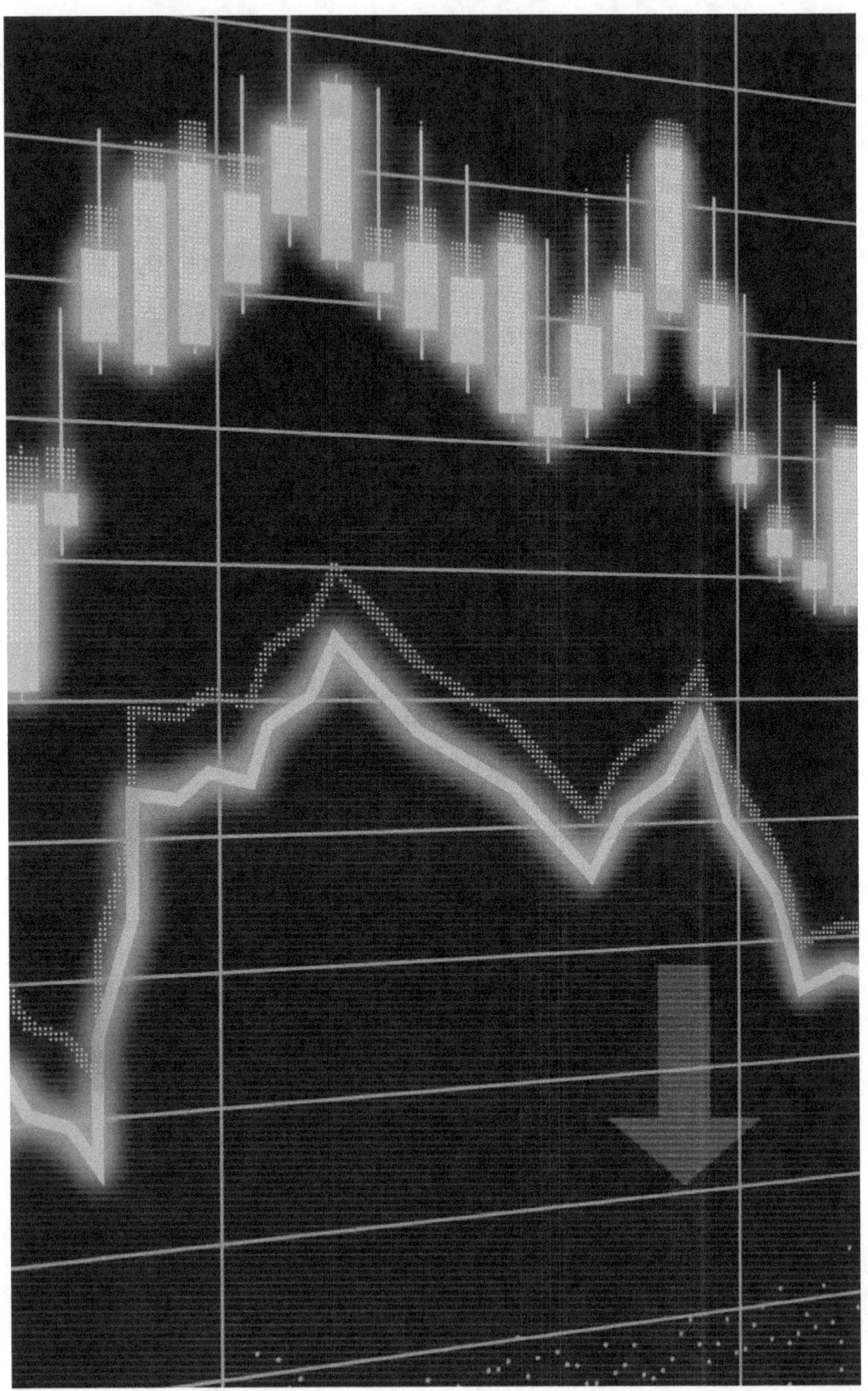

6. Analysis of Risks in AI Applications in Healthcare

In addition to the outlined opportunities associated with the integration of Artificial Intelligence in the medical sector, significant dimensions of risk emerge. This section takes a closer look at potential hazards related to the possible misuse of health data, misinterpretations, lack of transparency, and discriminatory influences.

Particular emphasis is placed on the transformation of the relationship between healthcare professionals and patients, raising the question of whether human empathy could potentially be displaced by algorithms.

6.1 Potential Misuse of Health Data

A prominent concern associated with the integration of Artificial Intelligence in healthcare is the previously mentioned data protection, conflicting with the need for training data. The risk of misuse of sensitive health data is particularly critical.

A study in the medical journal underscores significant concerns related to the security of personal health information. The increased integration of AI in medical decision-making processes makes the confidentiality of sensitive patient data more vulnerable to data breaches or unauthorized access.

This underscores the urgent need to implement robust security measures ensuring the confidentiality and integrity of health data.

The application of Artificial Intelligence entails two significant risks that must be acknowledged.

Firstly, while these algorithms statistically achieve excellent results or decisions in many scenarios, it does not imply infallibility. This issue, known as hallucination, can occur, especially in chatbots, due to insufficient data or weaknesses in the model's architecture and training data.

Despite advanced capabilities in synthesizing knowledge, pragmatics, and abstract thinking, models may struggle to maintain accuracy in complex inference tasks.

Secondly, machine learning approaches often operate as black boxes, meaning they cannot provide a clear explanation for why they arrive at a specific result. This is particularly problematic in sensitive areas such as human resources, where algorithms are used to make decisions about employees.

When an algorithm makes a selection based on behavioral profiles or applications without providing a clear explanation, it can not only pose difficulties in explaining the decision to applicants but also raise ethical concerns if certain parameters such as gender, skin color, or religion were involved. Artificial Neural Networks contribute to the lack of transparency in decision-making due to their opaque structure.

Moreover, biases, prejudices, and potential discrimination are frequently discussed risk factors. From data collection and training data stages, there is a risk of certain groups of people with specific characteristics being under- or overrepresented.
During model development, adjustments may be made in recursive loops, leading to further biases.

Lastly, the risk of discrimination exists in specific practical contexts if AI models are not carefully reviewed and adjusted for potential inequalities during application.

6.2 Restriction of Interaction between Healthcare Professionals and Patients

The implementation of Artificial Intelligence in healthcare brings about an evolutionary shift in the traditional relationship between healthcare professionals and patients, ranging from digital assistance systems to machine-driven decisions without human intervention.

This development not only raises ethical questions, particularly in areas where human interactions play a central role, but also replaces the previous empathy-oriented approach with a new understanding of roles.

For patients, this implies increased demands on health literacy, i.e., the ability to understand, evaluate, and apply health-related information. Studies from 2014 conducted by the scientific institute of AOK indicate that approximately 60% of respondents lack adequate prerequisites for health literacy. From a medical perspective, this necessitates addressing issues such as liability, responsibility, accountability, explicability, and legal certainty.

In the future, it will be crucial not only to explore technological potentials but also to understand the risks that could jeopardize the personal interaction between healthcare providers and patients, as well as compromise the fundamental principles of patient care.

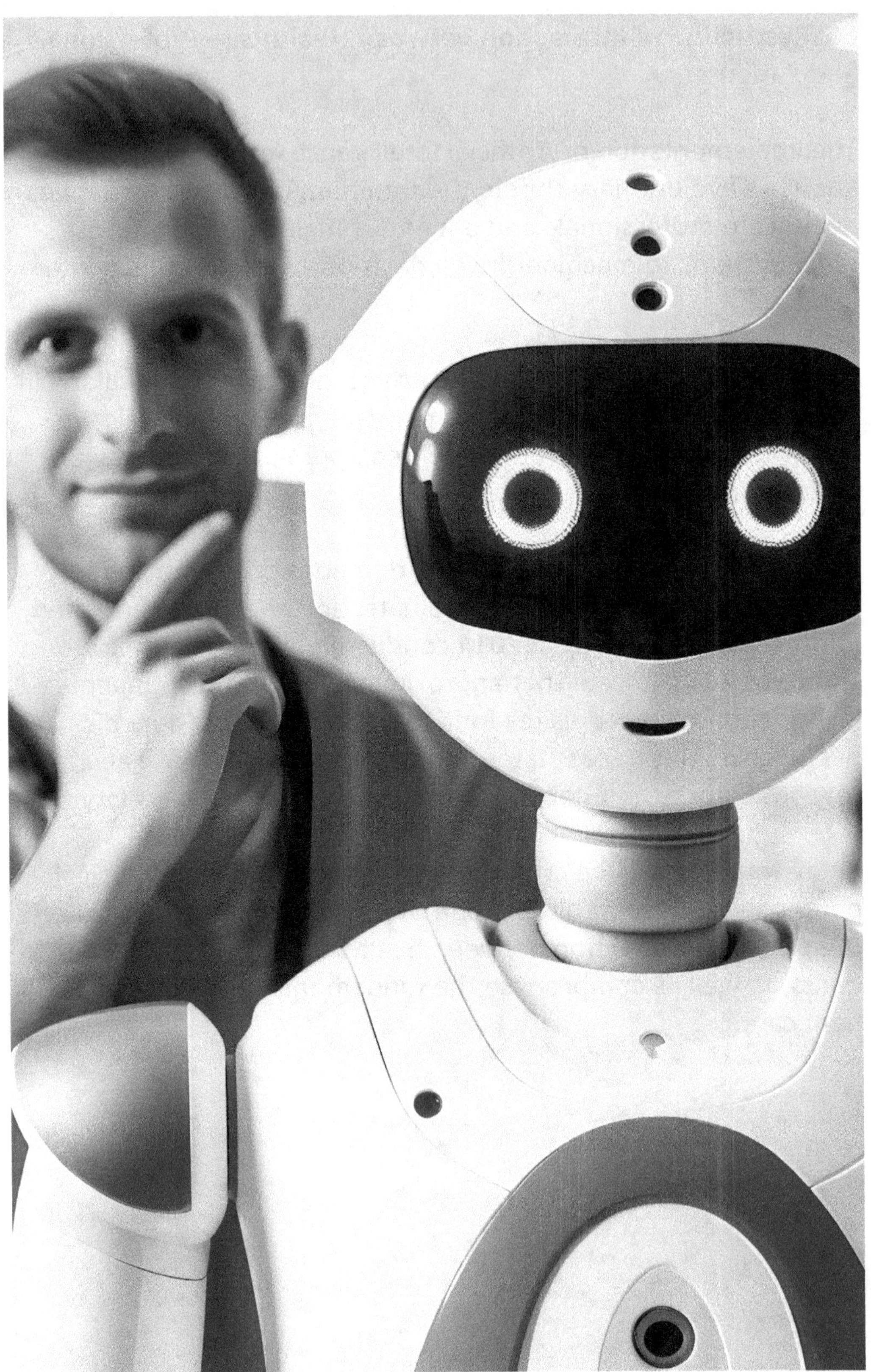

7. Conclusion and Outlook

The implementation of AI is considered a technological revolution that will transform all aspects of our lives. In healthcare, AI already plays a crucial role and will be a decisive factor in ensuring high-quality healthcare in the future. This progress requires not only technical prerequisites, such as high-quality medical datasets but also clear ethical and legal frameworks to instill trust in the technology and advance human rights-compliant and socially beneficial regulation of AI. Despite international efforts and expert committees, societal concerns persist, and the acceptance of AI depends on the perception of benefits and manageable risks.

To address this, involved companies must communicate more openly and become more transparent. Legislators are challenged to ensure data protection and create conditions for the approval, regulation, and liability of AI-based applications without hindering innovation. The processing and utilization of data will play a central role, and widespread access to digitalized medical information remains a challenge. The development of Big Data centers and the planned European Health Data Space aim to address this issue and improve access to research data. However, in Germany and the EU, the broad adoption of AI applications will occur gradually due to low technology adoption and stricter regulatory conditions.

Nevertheless, various application examples showcase the expected potential of such applications in healthcare. The use of AI promises significant benefits in medical research, administration, and care, including time savings, enhanced work quality, and more efficient resource utilization. Although some concepts may only be realizable in the medium term, short-term applications like medical chatbots and AI-supported diagnosis are already evident. AI will enhance medical care by assisting healthcare professionals in early disease detection.

The market for mobile health apps for health prevention is extensive, with numerous applications covering various health topics and mobile medical apps for diagnosis and disease prevention. In addressing health crises, AI will gain increasing importance, playing a central role in early detection, prediction, and containment of disease outbreaks. AI will also be increasingly used in virus analysis. Intelligent Big Data analyses are crucial in developing new pharmaceutical agents and understanding disease mechanisms, allowing for efficient identification of statistical correlations in extensive databases, expanding hypothesis testability, and playing a central role in cancer research and genomics. In drug development and clinical trials, AI optimizes the development cycle, shortens time-to-market, and enables efficient process improvements.

However, the integration of Artificial Intelligence in healthcare also poses risks, including data protection issues and the danger of algorithmic misinterpretation. The complex ethical challenge lies in balancing the protection of sensitive health data with the need for training data. Furthermore, the integration of AI in healthcare significantly alters the healthcare professional-patient relationship, from digital assistants to autonomous decisions. This raises ethical questions, requiring a thorough examination of liability and legal aspects to harness the benefits of AI without jeopardizing the fundamental principles of patient care. Clear regulatory standards and robust security measures are crucial to strengthen trust in the use of AI in healthcare.

In summary, Artificial Intelligence in healthcare offers the possibility to solve problems faster, more efficiently, and cost-effectively than human intelligence. This technology promises improved care, more precise diagnoses, and potential cost savings. However, the integration of AI should be done with strict adherence to ethical principles to fully leverage the potential of this technology while protecting the interests and rights of patients. New technologies and insights are continually introduced, and regulatory authorities and the healthcare community must keep pace. Research and discussion are crucial to ensure that the benefits of AI are utilized while minimizing associated risks.

The idea of a "Dr. AI" as part of medical care and risks associated with data handling may initially be alarming to many. Nevertheless, studies show that a basic trust in AI exists on both the side of patients and healthcare professionals. Through responsible use of AI, we can obtain more precise diagnoses, develop personalized therapies, and overall achieve a higher quality of medical care. With the right balance between technology and human expertise, it is ultimately possible to elevate medical care to a new level that enhances the well-being of patients.

About the Author:

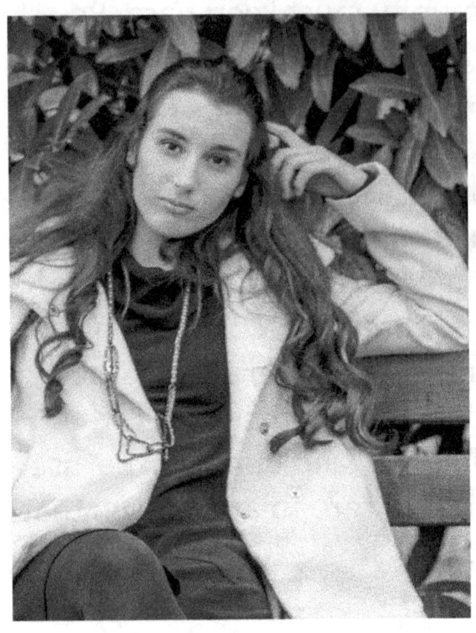

Michelle Gresbek, born in May 2000 in Erlangen, is a dedicated and highly qualified expert in the healthcare sector. This year, she will complete her Bachelor of Applied Science (BASc) in Health/Health Care Administration/Management at Alice Salomon University of Applied Sciences in Berlin. Throughout her studies, she acquired comprehensive knowledge of health administration and management with a focus on "Artificial Intelligence."

With her practical experience as a Medical Assistant, Michelle brings a solid foundation in medical care. She underwent extensive training, covering medical procedures, patient care, and administrative responsibilities at Ludwig Erhard Berufskolleg.

In addition to her successful professional career, Michelle Gresbek has excelled as an author. She has published several books, including "Natürliche Leberheilung" (Kindle-Ausgabe), "Tolle Rezepte zur natürlichen Leberheilung" (ISBN: 979-8838413291) und "Diabetes ist keine Sackgasse" (ISBN 79-8787914641).

The present book is also available in German, both as a paperback (ISBN 979-8879263268) and a hardcover edition (ISBN 979-8879267419).

These books reflect her passion for health topics and her commitment to sharing knowledge and practices in the healthcare sector.

Recommended Books (German):

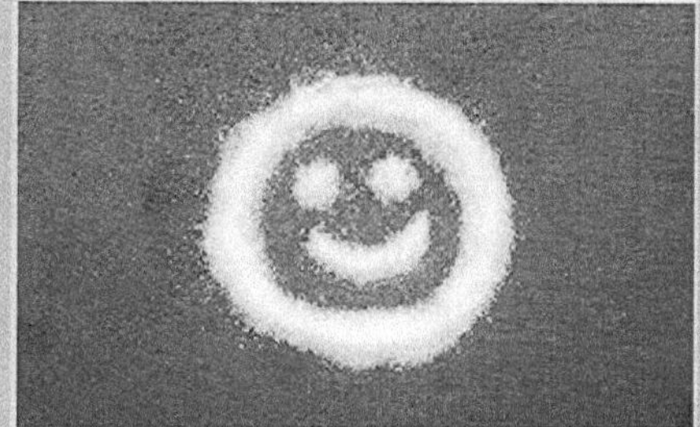

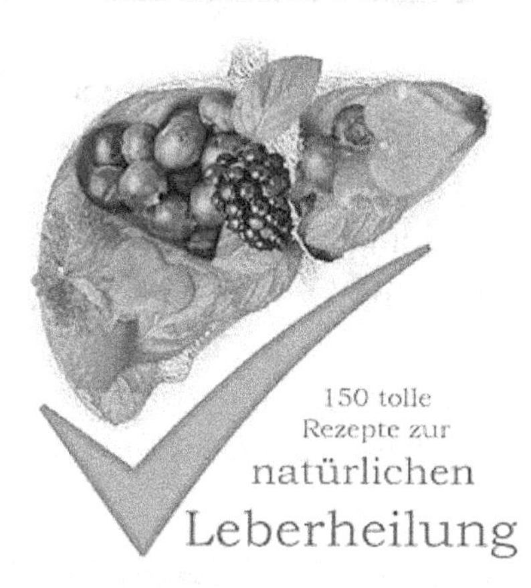

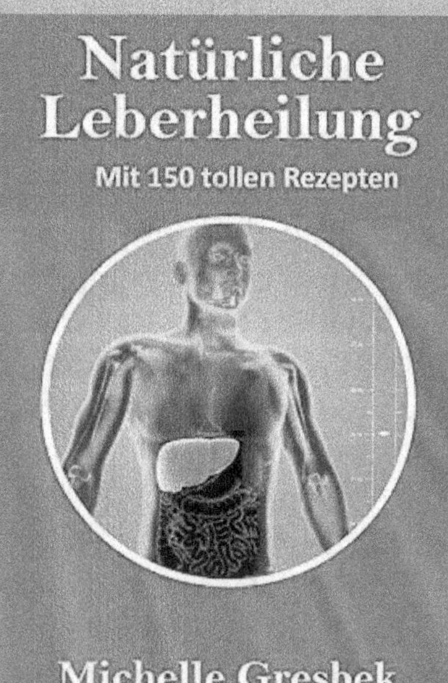

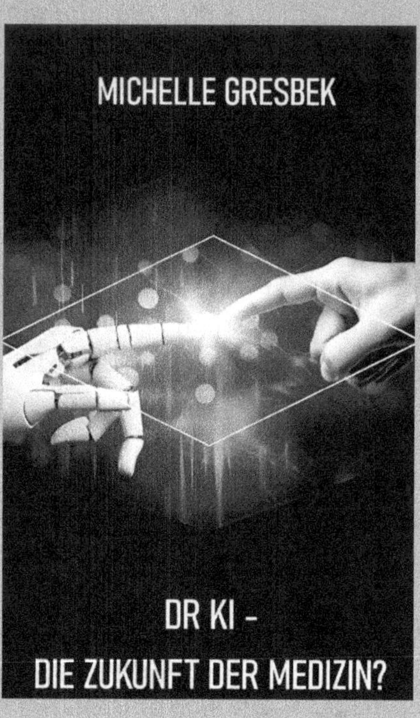

Bibliography

Aerzteblatt (2018) Künstliche Intelligenz für Ärzte und Patienten: „Googeln" war gestern Aerzteblatt.de. Abgerufen am 18.10.23 von https://www.aerzteblatt.de/archiv/198854/Kuenstliche-Intelligenz-fuer-Aerzte-und-Patienten-Googeln-war-gestern

Aerzteblatt (2020) Künstliche Intelligenz: Patienten im Fokus Aerzteblatt.de. Abgerufen am 24.10.23 von https://www.aerzteblatt.de/archiv/216998/Kuenstliche-Intelligenz-Patienten-im-Fokus

Airamed (2023) Künstliche Intelligenz macht Neuroradiologie messbar Airamed. Abgerufen am 01.11.23 von https://www.airamed.de/de/startseite

Barkhausen, B. (2023) Künstliche Intelligenz: Google-CEO Sundar Pichai spricht ernste Warnung aus Gründerszene. Abgerufen am 02.10.23 von https://www.businessinsider.de/gruenderszene/business/google-sundar-pichai-ki-warnung/

Barton, M.-C. & Pöppelbuß, J. (2022) Prinzipien für die ethische Nutzung künstlicher Intelligenz Springer Verlag. Abgerufen am 18.09.23 von https://link.springer.com/content/pdf/10.1365/s40702-022-00850-3.pdf

Bayer, M. (2023) US-Präsident Biden will KI stärker regulieren Computerwoche Voice of Digital. Abgerufen am 13.11.23 von https://www.computerwoche.de/a/us-praesident-biden-will-ki-staerker-regulieren,3615556

Benaich, N. & Air Street Captial (2023) AI for science: medicine is growing fastest but mathematics captures the most attention State of AI Report. Abgerufen am 07.11.23 von https://www.stateof.ai/

Bommasani, R. et al. (2023) The Foundation Model Transparency Index Center for Research on Foundation Models. Abgerufen am 10.10.23 von https://crfm.stanford.edu/fmti/

Bradshaw, J. C. (2023) The ChatGPT Era: Artificial Intelligence in Emergency Medicine Annals of Emergency Medicine. Abgerufen am 22.10.23 von https://www.annemergmed.com/article/S0196-0644(23)00035-5/fulltext

Bratan, T. (2023) Künstliche Intelligenz im Gesundheitsbereich: Ein Überblick Fraunhofer Institut. Abgerufen am 14.09.23 von https://www.isi.fraunhofer.de/de/blog/2023/kuenstliche-intelligenz-im-gesundheitsbereich.html

Bundesfinanzministerium (2018) Strategie Künstliche Intelligenz Bundesfinanzministerium. Abgerufen am 06.10.23 von https://www.bundesfinanzministerium.de/Content/DE/Downloads/Digitalisierung/2018-11-15-Strategie-zur-Kuenstlichen-Intelligenz.pdf?__blob=publicationFile S. 5

Bundesministerium für Bildung und Forschung (2020) Künstliche Intelligenz für Krebsbehandlung nutzen Pressemitteilung BMBF. Abgerufen am 08.10.23 von https://www.bmbf.de/bmbf/shareddocs/downloads/files/2020-03-05_027-

pm-cancer-scout.pdf?__blob=publicationFile&v=1

Bünte, C. (2022) Künstliche Intelligenz – Ein Überblick über die aktuelle und zukünftige Bedeutung von KI in der Wirtschaft und im Gesundheitswesen in Europa Springer Verlag. Abgerufen am 07.09.23 von https://link.springer.com/chapter/10.1007/978-3-658-33597-7_3

Büttner, M. (2022) KI hilft chronisch Erkrankten digitales Hessen. Abgerufen am 18.10.23 von https://digitales.hessen.de/presse/ki-hilft-chronisch-erkrankten

Buxmann, P. & Schmidt, H. (2018) Grundlagen der Künstlichen Intelligenz und des Maschinellen Lernens Springer Verlag. Abgerufen am 16.09.23 von https://link.springer.com/chapter/10.1007/978-3-662-57568-0_1

Carlos (2023) ChatGPT: Die wichtigsten Statistiken und Daten (02/2023) Finantio. Abgerufen am 13.10.22 von https://finantio.de/wissen/chatgpt-statistiken/

Deloitte (2022) Fueling the AI transformation Four key actions powering widespread value from AI, right now in Germany Deloitte's State of AI in the Enterprise. Abgerufen am 14.11.23 von https://www2.deloitte.com/us/en/pages/consulting/articles/state-of-ai-2022.html

Dohrmann, M. & Knupfmann, S. (2022) KÜNSTLICHE INTELLIGENZ GESUNDHEITSSEKTOR Handelsblatt Research Institute. Abgerufen am 10.09.23 von https://veranstaltungen.handelsblatt.com/health-circle/wp-content/uploads/2022/10/Health_Circle_KI-im-Gesundheitssektor.pdf

Döpfner, M. (2016) Mark Zuckerberg im Interview: „Die Furcht vor künstlicher Intelligenz ist eher hysterisch" Business Insider. Abgerufen am 26.10.23 von https://www.businessinsider.de/tech/mark-zuckerberg-im-interview-die-furcht-vor-kuenstlicher-intelligenz-ist-eher-hysterisch/

Eckermann, I. M. (2020) Wie medizinische Wearables und Fitness-Tracker unsere Gesundheit verändern dara4life. Abgerufen am 08.09.23 von https://www.data4life.care/de/bibliothek/journal/medizinische-wearables-und-fitness-tracker/

Europäisches Parlament (2023) KI-Gesetz: erste Regulierung der künstlichen Intelligenz Europäisches Parlament. Abgerufen am 16.11.23 von https://www.europarl.europa.eu/news/de/headlines/society/20230601STO93804/ki-gesetz-erste-regulierung-der-kunstlichen-intelligenz

Fraunhofer Gesellschaft (2022) Smartphone-App und KI-Software beschleunigen Erkennung von Hautkrebs Fraunhofer Gesellschaft. Abgerufen am 14.09.23 von https://www.fraunhofer.de/de/presse/presseinformationen/2022/februar-2022/smartphone-app-und-ki-software-beschleunigen-erkennung-von-hautkrebs.html

Fraunhofer-Institut (2023) Künstliche Intelligenz (KI) und maschinelles Lernen IKS Fraunhofer. Abgerufen am 14.09.23 von https://www.iks.fraunhofer.de/de/themen/kuenstliche-intelligenz.html

Fraunhofer Magazin (2023) KI in der Medizin Fraunhofer. Abgerufen am 14.09.23 von https://www.fraunhofer.de/de/forschung/aktuelles-aus-der-forschung/ki-in-der-medizin.html

Geeksforgeeks (2023) What is Machine Learning? Geeksforgeeks. Abgerufen am 09.10.23 von https://www.geeksforgeeks.org/what-is-machine-learning/

Gillissen, A. (2019) Künstliche Intelligenz schlägt Lungenärzte Springer Verlag. Abgerufen am 10.09.23 von https://link.springer.com/article/10.1007/s15006-019-0955-0

Gov.uk (2023) Policy paper: Chair's Summary of the AI Safety Summit 2023, Bletchley Park Gov.uk. Abgerufen am 24.11.23 von https://www.gov.uk/government/publications/ai-safety-summit-2023-chairs-statement-2-november/chairs-summary-of-the-ai-safety-summit-2023-bletchley-park#contents

Heaven, D. W. (2023) Generative KI: Die Geschichte hinter ChatGPT heise online. Abgerufen am 17.10.23 von https://www.heise.de/hintergrund/Generative-KI-Die-Geschichte-hinter-ChatGPT-8243968.html

Heise Medien (2023) Wie künstliche Intelligenz bei der Erkennung, Abwehr und Eindämmung von COVID-19 helfen kann. Heise Business Service. Abgerufen am 04.11.23 von https://business-services.heise.de/specials/moderne-it-infrastruktur/home/beitrag/ki-im-kampf-gegen-corona-3963

Jones, S. (2023) Wie kann KI zur Bewältigung von Herausforderungen im Bereich der öffentlichen Gesundheit eingesetzt werden? Webmedy. Abgerufen am 02.11.23 von https://webmedy.com/blog/de/ai-public-health/

Jorzig, A. & Sarangi, F. (2020) Digitalisierung im Gesundheitswesen Springer Verlag. Abgerufen am 19.10.23 von https://www.springerprofessional.de/digitalisierung-im-gesundheitswesen/18006568

Kaplan, A. & Haenlein, M. (2019) Siri, Siri, in my hand: Who's the fairest in the land? On the interpretations, illustrations, and implications of artificial intelligence Science Direct. Abgerufen am 08.09.23 von https://www.sciencedirect.com/science/article/abs/pii/S0007681318301393?via%3Dihub S. 3

Kolpatzik, K. et al. (2020) DIGITALE GESUNDHEITSKOMPETENZ AOK. Abgerufen am 19.11.23 von https://aok-bv.de/imperia/md/aokbv/gesundheitskompetenz/studienbericht_digitale_gk_web.pdf

König, H., et al. (2021) Künstliche Intelligenz in der genomischen Medizin – Potentiale und Handlungsbedarf Policy Brief Fraunhofer ISI. Abgerufen am 15.09.23 von https://www.isi.fraunhofer.de/content/dam/isi/dokumente/cct/2021/Policy%20Brief%202021_KI%20in%20der%20genomischen%20Medizin.pdf

Lauterbach, A. (2022) Mit KI das Gesundheitswesen verändern Springer Verlag. Abgerufen am 01.10.23 von https://link.springer.com/chapter/10.1007/978-3-658-33597-7_4

Liu et al. (2023) Exposing Attention Glitches with Flip-Flop Language

Modeling Cornell University. Abgerufen am 21.11.23 von https://arxiv.org/abs/2306.00946

Madoff, L & Brownstein, J. (2010) ProMED and HealthMap: Collaboration to improve emerging disease surveillance International Journal of Infectious Diseases. Abgerufen am 15.11.23 von https://www.ijidonline.com/article/S1201-9712(10)01938-7/fulltext

McKinsey (2017) Künstliche Intelligenz wird zum Wachstumsmotor für deutsche Industrie McKinsey & Company. Abgerufen am 09.10.23 von https://www.mckinsey.com/de/news/presse/kunstliche-intelligenz-wird-zum-wachstumsmotor-fur-deutsche-industrie

Medizinio (2021) Künstliche Intelligenz – Die Zukunft der Medizin? Medizinio der Medizintechnikmarkt. Abgerufen am 18.09.23 von https://www.medizintechnikmarkt.de/blog/ki-medizin

Merz, D. & Hübner, J. (2022) Bessere Medizin? Künstliche Intelligenz verantwortlich gestalten Springer Verlag. Abgerufen am 08.09.23 von https://link.springer.com/chapter/10.1007/978-3-658-33597-7_11

Mester, B. A. (2018) Datenschutzrechtliche Herausforderung der „Künstlichen Intelligenz" (KI) Springer Verlag. Abgerufen am 17.10.23 von https://link.springer.com/content/pdf/10.1007/s11623-018-0993-2.pdf

NFDI4Health (2023) Nationale Forschungsdateninfrastruktur für personenbezogene Gesundheitsdaten NFDI4Health. Abgerufen am 14.10.23 von https://www.nfdi4health.de/

Palder, K. (2023) Künstliche Intelligenz im Kampf gegen den Krebs Siemens Healthineers. Abgerufen am 22.10.23 von https://www.siemens-healthineers.com/deu/perspectives/AI-cancer-care

Pechmann, L. et al. (2022) Regulatorische Anforderungen an Lösungen der künstlichen Intelligenz im Gesundheitswesen Springer Verlag. Abgerufen am 14.09.23 von https://link.springer.com/chapter/10.1007/978-3-658-33597-7_8

Rasche, C. & Brehmer, N. (2022) KI-Implementierungsoptionen in dateninflationären Versorgungsnetzen: Von der abstrakten Vision zur konkreten Wertschöpfungstransformation Springer Verlag. Abgerufen am 08.10.23 von https://link.springer.com/chapter/10.1007/978-3-658-33597-7_9

Rasche, C. et al. (2022) Künstliche Intelligenz im Gesundheitswesen als Kernkompetenz? Status quo, Entwicklungslinien und disruptives Potenzial Springer Verlag. Abgerufen am 24.10.23 von https://link.springer.com/chapter/10.1007/978-3-658-33597-7_2

Reardon, S. (2023) AI Chatbots Can Diagnose Medical Conditions at Home. How Good Are They? SCIAM. Abgerufen am 02.11.23 von https://www.scientificamerican.com/article/ai-chatbots-can-diagnose-medical-conditions-at-home-how-good-are-they/

Ruschemeier, H. (2023) Regulierung von KI bpb. Abgerufen am 21.11.23 von https://www.bpb.de/shop/zeitschriften/apuz/kuenstliche-intelligenz-2023/541498/regulierung-von-ki/

Schirmer, H. (2022) Artificial Intelligence in Healthcare American Journal of Biomedical Science & Research. Abgerufen am 04.09.23 von Prof. Dr. Schirmer

Schirmer, H. (2022) Chancen und Grenzen der Digitalisierung im Gesundheitswesen zur nachhaltigen Förderung der Bevölkerungsgesundheit in Deutschland Springer Verlag. Abgerufen am 04.09.23 von https://link.springer.com/chapter/10.1007/978-3-658-36484-7_12

Schmidt, T. & Winter, J. (2022) Künstliche Intelligenz in Prozessen des Gesundheitswesens – Chancen und Risiken am Beispiel der akuten Schlaganfallbehandlung Springer Verlag. Abgerufen am 08.09.23 von https://link.springer.com/chapter/10.1007/978-3-658-33597-7_21

Schneeweiss, S. (2023) Von Real-World-Daten zur Real-World-Evidenz: eine praktische Anleitung Springer Verlag. Abgerufen am 04.11.23 von https://link.springer.com/article/10.1007/s11553-023-01026-7

Schneider, I. (2021) KI in der Medizin Zeitschrift für medizinische Ethik. Abgerufen am 28.11.23 von https://www.inf.uni-hamburg.de/en/inst/ab/eit/files/zfme2021-03-schneider-ki-diskriminierung-web-end.pdf

Schulzki-Haddouti, C. (2023) Digital Health: MedPaLM im Medizinertest auf Augenhöhe heise online. Abgerufen am 26.10.23 von https://www.heise.de/news/Digital-Health-Med-PaLM-im-Medizinertest-auf-Augenhoehe-9214542.html

Schweighöfer, S. C. & Pfannstiel, M. A. (2022) Künstliche Intelligenz im Entwicklungsprozess von Medikamenten in der Pharmaindustrie Springer Verlag. Abgerufen am 13.10.23 von https://link.springer.com/chapter/10.1007/978-3-658-33597-7_6

Schwenke, T. (2023) KI & Datenschutz – Checkliste für den Einsatz künstlicher Intelligenz Datenschutz – Generator. Abgerufen am 14.10.23 von https://datenschutz-generator.de/ki-datenschutz/

Sciencelu (2023) Studie: ChatGPT bei Diagnose in der Notaufnahme so gut wie Ärzte Sciencelu. Abgerufen am 15.09.23 von https://www.science.lu/de/studie-chatgpt-bei-diagnose-der-notaufnahme-so-gut-wie-aerzte

Sree, S. V., et al. (2020) An introduction to the Cyrcadia Breast Monitor: A wearable breast health monitoring device Pubmed Verlag. Abgerufen am 21.10.23 von https://pubmed.ncbi.nlm.nih.gov/33007593/

Stallkamp, J., et al. (2022) KI-Systeme für die nächste Medizintechnikgeneration Springer Verlag. Abgerufen am 13.10.23 von https://link.springer.com/chapter/10.1007/978-3-658-33597-7_7

Teipel, S. (2019) MRT-Untersuchung nur bei kognitiven Einschränkungen Alzheimer Forschung Initiative e.V. Abgerufen am 18.10.23 von https://www.alzheimer-forschung.de/aktuelles/meldung/mrt-untersuchung-nur-bei-kogni-

tiven-einschraenkungen/
The White House (2023) Executive Order on the Safe, Secure, and Trustworthy Development and Use of Artificial Intelligence The White House.
Abgerufen am 13.11.23 von https://www.whitehouse.gov/briefing-room/pres-
idential-actions/2023/10/30/executive-order-on-the-safe-secure-and-trust-
worthy-development-and-use-of-artificial-intelligence/
Torsten, R. (2023) Großbritannien: Britischer Premierminister Sunak warnt
vor Risiken Künstlicher Intelligenz Handelsblatt. Abgerufen am 19.11.23
von https://www.handelsblatt.com/politik/international/grossbritan-
nien-britischer-premierminister-sunak-warnt-vor-risiken-kuenstlicher-intelli-
genz/29467428.html
Tudor Car et al. (2020) Conversational Agents in Health Care: Scoping Review
and Conceptual Analysis Research Gate. Abgerufen am 16.10.23 von https://
www.researchgate.net/publication/343519716_Conversational_Agents_in_
Health_Care_Scoping_Review_and_Conceptual_Analysis
UNESCO (2023) UNESCO-Empfehlung zur Ethik der Künstlichen Intelligenz
in Deutschland UNESCO. Abgerufen am 14.11.23 von https://www.unesco.de/
wissen/wissenschaft/ethik-und-philosophie/studie-umsetzung-ki-ethik-emp-
fehlung
Weber, N. (2023) ChatGPT wird mit GPT-4 Turbo und seinem Zugriff auf
Informationen ab 2023 weniger veraltet sein Futuriq. Abgerufen am 08.10.23
von https://futuriq.de/2023/11/chatgpt/chatgpt-wird-mit-gpt-4-turbo-und-
seinem-zugriff-auf-informationen-ab-2023-weniger-veraltet-sein/130863/
Wenz, F. & Ebener, S. (2023) Anwendungen künstlicher Intelligenz in der
Onkologie: Möglichkeiten, Machbarkeit und regulatorische Herausforderungen Springer Verlag. Abgerufen am 15.11.23 von https://link.springer.com/
article/10.1007/s00761-023-01428-4
Wess, S. (2018) Mit Künstlicher Intelligenz immer die richtigen Entschei-
dungen treffen Springer Verlag. Abgerufen am 26.10.23 von https://link.
springer.com/chapter/10.1007/978-3-662-57568-0_9